AF711892

DBT NEXT STEPS CLINICIAN'S MANUAL

Also Available

FOR PROFESSIONALS

Cognitive-Behavioral Treatment of Borderline Personality Disorder
Marsha M. Linehan

DBT Skills Training Handouts and Worksheets, Revised Edition
Marsha M. Linehan

DBT Skills Training Manual, Revised Edition
Marsha M. Linehan

DBT Teams: Development and Practice
Jennifer H. R. Sayrs and Marsha M. Linehan

Dialectical Behavior Therapy with Suicidal Adolescents
Alec L. Miller, Jill H. Rathus, and Marsha M. Linehan

Mindfulness and Acceptance: Expanding the Cognitive-Behavioral Tradition
Edited by Steven C. Hayes, Victoria M. Follette, and Marsha M. Linehan

FOR GENERAL READERS

Coping with Cancer: DBT Skills to Manage Your Emotions—and Balance Uncertainty with Hope
Elizabeth Cohn Stuntz and Marsha M. Linehan

DBT Next Steps Clinician's Manual

Building a Life Worth Living

Katherine Anne Comtois
Adam Carmel
Marsha M. Linehan

THE GUILFORD PRESS
New York London

A Division of Guilford Publications, Inc.
www.guilford.com

Printed in the United States of America

This book is printed on acid-free paper.

For product and safety concerns within the EU, please contact *GPSR@taylorandfrancis.com*, Taylor & Francis Verlag GmbH, Kaufingerstraße 24, 80331 München, Germany.

Last digit is print number: 9 8 7 6 5 4 3 2 1

The authors have checked with sources believed to be reliable in their efforts to provide information that is complete and generally in accord with the standards of practice that are accepted at the time of publication. However, in view of the possibility of human error or changes in behavioral, mental health, or medical sciences, neither the authors, nor the editor and publisher, nor any other party who has been involved in the preparation or publication of this work warrants that the information contained herein is in every respect accurate or complete, and they are not responsible for any errors or omissions or the results obtained from the use of such information. Readers are encouraged to confirm the information contained in this book with other sources.

Library of Congress Cataloging-in-Publication Data is available from the publisher.

ISBN 978-1-4625-5811-7 (paperback) ISBN 978-1-4625-5812-4 (hardcover)

About the Authors

Katherine Anne Comtois, PhD, MPH, is Professor in the Department of Psychiatry and Behavioral Sciences and Adjunct Professor in the Department of Psychology at the University of Washington. She was a research therapist and co-investigator with Marsha Linehan on her clinical trials from 1994 to 2006 and Director of the DBT program at Harborview Mental Health and Addiction Services from 1996 to 2019. She now leads the DBT clinic and training program at the University of Washington Medical Center Outpatient Psychiatry Clinic. Dr. Comtois provides training and consultation on DBT Next Steps and the DBT-ACES program through the University of Washington. In addition, Dr. Comtois provides training and consultation in standard DBT internationally as an independent contractor with Treatment Implementation Collaborative LLC.

Adam Carmel, PhD, is Clinical Professor in the Department of Psychiatry and Behavioral Sciences at the University of Washington. He is Codirector of the Annual Comprehensive DBT Training program in the Department of Psychiatry and Behavioral Sciences at the University of Washington. He was previously Director of the Massachusetts Mental Health Center's DBT program operated by the Massachusetts Department of Mental Health. Dr. Carmel was previously Clinical Assistant Professor in the Department of Psychology at the University of Washington, where he taught DBT in the Behavioral Research and Therapy Clinics under the direction of Marsha Linehan.

Marsha M. Linehan, PhD, ABPP, the developer of Dialectical Behavior Therapy (DBT), is Professor Emeritus of Psychology and Director Emeritus of the Behavioral Research and Therapy Clinics at the University of Washington. Before retiring in 2019, she devoted her career to developing and evaluating evidence-based treatments for populations with high suicide risk and multiple, severe mental disorders. Dr. Linehan is the 2025 recipient of the Lifetime

Achievement Award from the American Foundation for Suicide Prevention. Her contributions to suicide research and clinical psychology research have also been recognized with the University of Louisville Grawemeyer Award for Psychology, the Career/Lifetime Achievement Award from the Association for Behavioral and Cognitive Therapies, the Gold Medal Award for Life Achievement in the Application of Psychology from the American Psychological Foundation, and the James McKeen Cattell Award from the Association for Psychological Science. In her honor, the American Association of Suicidology created the Marsha Linehan Award for Outstanding Research in the Treatment of Suicidal Behavior. Dr. Linehan was featured in *TIME Great Scientists: The Geniuses and Visionaries Who Transformed Our World*. She is founder of the Linehan Institute and is a Zen master.

Acknowledgments

Many people came together over 20 years to make this book a reality. We would like to first acknowledge Marsha M. Linehan, PhD, without whose brilliance, creativity, and perseverance there would be no DBT to adapt. In addition, it is through her critical thinking that the fuzzy concepts and strategies that come from running and developing a program simultaneously became clear and precise in this book.

We would like to acknowledge the many partners who were critical to DBT Next Steps success. Hugh Armstrong, PhD, was the first person to take a chance on implementing DBT when it was still in its formative stages and developed the Harborview DBT Program. JoAnn Marsden, BA RT, was the consistent lead of Harborview DBT for 30 years. Their support of the big ideas of Kate Comtois, when she was a young psychologist, set the stage and provided the platform for this work. We would like to thank JoAnn as well as Marty Hoiness, MD; Lynn Elwood, LMHC; Kristina Campbell, LMHC; Cristina Mullen, LICSW; Penni Brinkerhoff, LMHC; Wayne Smith, PhD; Jenna Melman, LICSW; Mike McDonell, PhD; and Britt Alvy, LICSW from the Harborview DBT Program for their wisdom and insights in developing and implementing DBT–Accepting the Challenges of Employment and Self-Sufficiency (DBT-ACES) comprehensive program over the years. Glenette Olvera, MSW; Richard Ries, MD; Peter Roy-Byrne, MD; and other members of the HMHAS leadership have provided not only ongoing support to DBT at Harborview but also specific encouragement to the DBT team for treatment development and innovation, including DBT-ACES. Lynn McFarr, PhD; Lisa Bolden, PsyD; and others at the Harbor–UCLA DBT-ACES program and Klaus and Stephanie Höeschel in the German DBT-ACES program have been amazing partners and shared critical wisdom. The National Institute of Mental Health and the Catherine Wilkins Foundation provided critical financial support allowing us to evaluate and improve the program. We also want to thank our editor, Kitty Moore, who made DBT Next Steps possible. She saw the potential for DBT Next Steps and collaborated with us to transform our DBT-ACES treatment manuals for research into much stronger and more useful books.

And, of course, DBT Next Steps would not exist if the Harborview DBT-ACES clients had not stepped up to every challenge set before them. Together with us, they showed the courage to try for more and more ambitious employment, college, and self-sufficiency. They have surely accepted this challenge. It has been and still is a joy and a privilege to witness.

Finally, none of this could happen without the support of our families. Kate is deeply grateful to her wife, Teresa, who has been the rock of support—both emotionally and with the countless day-to-day demands—that made all of this possible, and to her parents, her son, Courtney, and her sister, Liza, who have always supported her hopes and dreams. Adam thanks his family, who have provided years of love and support, including his husband, Ben; his son, Nathan; and all the friends and colleagues who offered encouragement during the process of writing this book. And finally, thank you, Geri, for your help and support in making this book a reality for all of us.

Brief Contents

Extended Contents

PART I
SETTING THE STAGE

PART II
DBT NEXT STEPS STRATEGIES

PART III
INTEGRATING DBT NEXT STEPS INTO A COMPREHENSIVE DBT-ACES PROGRAM

PART IV
THE DBT-ACES SKILLS CURRICULUM

DBT NEXT STEPS CLINICIAN'S MANUAL

PART I

SETTING THE STAGE

CHAPTER 1

What Is Beyond the Crisis?

Development of DBT Next Steps

In 1992, Kate Comtois came to what is now called Harborview Mental Health and Addiction Services (HMHAS) for a postdoctoral fellowship with Hugh Armstrong, PhD. HMHAS is a public mental health center at Harborview Medical Center, which is owned by King County and managed by the University of Washington. In the late 1980s, the HMHAS Life Skills program was the first clinic to implement Dialectical Behavior Therapy (DBT) outside of Marsha Linehan's research clinic. When Kate arrived to assume her fellowship, Hugh assigned her the role of co-leader in the DBT skills-training group and gave her a copy of the prepublished DBT manual. (It was mimeographed—who is old enough to remember the smell of mimeograph paper and turning the crank to make the copies?) Kate discovered a love for DBT, particularly with suicidal clients, and was delighted by the opportunity late in her fellowship to work with Marsha Linehan as a screener for her new DBT clinical trials funded by the National Institute of Mental Health (NIMH) and the National Institute on Drug Abuse (NIDA) at the Behavioral Research and Therapy Clinics (BRTC). Harborview and the University of Washington decided to keep Kate on as faculty and, upon Hugh's retirement in 1996, asked her to take over directorship of the DBT program. She also became Marsha's associate director for BRTC.

As the Harborview DBT program graduated DBT clients over the 1990s, we were happy to see them move beyond suicidal coping to a stable life outside of the hospital. Kate and her team found that the outcomes for psychiatrically disabled individuals with severe and chronic borderline personality disorder (BPD) were comparable to the research trials (Comtois, Elwood, et al., 2007). However, as successful as we were in preventing suicidal behavior and associated emergency room and inpatient psychiatric admissions, our patients remained at the mental health center without structured activity such as work or school and continued to be dependent on the public mental health system. We tried adding a second year of DBT, but that didn't change outcomes very much and the DBT team was feeling a bit stuck. Then in 1999, the Harborview DBT team lost two graduates of our 2-year DBT program to suicide and enough was enough. We had to find a solution—we were working too hard, and the clients were working too hard, not to have greater recovery and quality of life.

We looked at options for other evidence-based treatments for employment such as Supported Employment (Blum et al., 2008; Cook et al., 2005; Drake et al., 1999; Markowitz et al., 2007) and Assertive Community Treatment (Drake & Deegan, 2008; Gold et al., 2004, 2006; Horvitz-Lennon et al., 2009), versions of which were also being implemented at HMHAS. But these interventions were not a good fit for individuals with BPD (Chanen et al., 2020; Swenson et al., 2002; Weisbrod, 1983) and did not share our goal of living wage employment and being able to leave the public mental health system. So, by trial and error of different strategies from DBT and elsewhere, and with ongoing consultation with Marsha and funding from the Catherine Wilkins Foundation and NIMH, we developed a new skills-training curriculum and adaptations to individual therapy focused primarily on contingency management and exposure to help clients take the next step in DBT.

Working in a public mental health agency funded by public insurance (called Medicare and Medicaid in the United States), clients, and we, were forced to deal with the challenges of getting off psychiatric disability and living outside of the social service system. Public mental health clients are generally told not to work too many hours or make too much money, so they don't risk their disability benefits, and many of these clients have experienced homelessness. Working enough to end disability payments means depending entirely on one's own ability to work, and if you lose your job, you risk having to move back with family or being homeless. For these and other reasons, clients often experience an increase in symptoms and substantial distress as they approach applying for, beginning, or changing employment. This often led us, as it does most vocational programs, to back off and stabilize symptoms before re-approaching employment. And then the process would repeat itself in a classic approach–avoid scenario. However, when the right contingencies are in place and DBT clients practice exposure by applying for jobs and start working, they generally find that after a few weeks of building up "work stamina," working is quite manageable. In fact, many clients have noted it is less stressful than being disabled.

It was through the process of helping clients persevere and successfully work or go to college that we became true converts to the behavioral adage that "Contingencies Create Capabilities." Cindy Sanderson, PhD, who was running a DBT program in New York, told us they required employment for clients to stay in their program beyond a certain point; otherwise, they had to drop out. This was a breakthrough idea for us. With Marsha's help to stay dialectical and ensure validation and reinforcement for progress by changing this from ending therapy to a "therapy vacation," we developed contingencies for "Work as Therapy" and career activities to make it easier for clients to achieve this big lift. This led us to our original program name: Accepting the Challenges of Employment and Self-Sufficiency, or DBT-ACES. DBT-ACES skills and strategies embody both acceptance of how things are now, while challenging clients to make crucial changes to achieve their ambitions.

Once we thought we had the DBT-ACES program mostly developed and had some pre–post pilot data showing success (Comtois et al., 2010), we obtained an NIMH treatment development grant from 2007 to 2010 to develop a manual and evaluate the results of a second pilot test. This grant allowed us to become more systematic. Kate and teammates from the Harborview DBT team met with Marsha regularly as part of this grant to examine each part of the program to be sure it was internally consistent as well as consistent with DBT. And, of course, because of Marsha, lots of creative and effective ideas got incorporated. We helped two DBT teams—at Harbor–UCLA and in Lengerich, Germany—implement DBT-ACES. Their experience with DBT-ACES further clarified and improved the program.

Adam Carmel joined us in the 2010s, when we expanded the reach of DBT-ACES from clients on state and federal psychiatric disability programs to those whose disability is provided by their employer or who are supported by their family. We have found that the core DBT issues are very similar for clients unable to work and fend for themselves whether they are rich or poor and did not require any adaptation to DBT-ACES. In concert with the Harbor–UCLA and German programs, Kate and Adam were able to replicate the pre–post findings of our original study with this expanded version of DBT-ACES across three sites (Comtois et al., 2020).

In 2018, Kate stopped leading our DBT-ACES skills group (a wrenching step after almost 20 years!) to be sure that we had a clinician's guide that worked without her in the room. Under Adam's leadership, the skills manual was shortened and revised based on notes taken from observing Kate teach, then observing the teaching of naive group leaders at Harborview and Harbor–UCLA. The final version of these new DBT skills is described in Part IV through detailed lesson plans and captured in our companion book for clients, *DBT Next Steps Skills Handouts.*

Since Marsha's retirement, Kate and Adam have expanded the focus beyond a comprehensive DBT-ACES program to more general principles on how to make a successful transition from DBT for acute and pervasive crisis behaviors (tearing your life down) to achieving "life worth living goals" (building something new and lasting). DBT Next Steps addresses a key challenge of DBT: The farther you get down the DBT hierarchy—past suicidal behavior and therapy-interfering behavior (TIB) and squarely into quality-of-life (QOL)-interfering behavior where a life worth living is built—the less the DBT manual can help you for three reasons. First, Marsha presumed a lot of experience and expertise with cognitive-behavioral therapy (CBT) that most therapists don't have (e.g., out of 523 pages of text in the DBT manual, only 36 pages—7%—are devoted to contingency management and 15 pages—3%—to exposure). Second, Marsha's research focused on highly suicidal or opiate-addicted clients in 1 year of treatment. In that time, few clients moved much farther than a first step in QOL-interfering behavior, and usually this targeted not tearing your life down (e.g., substance use, anxiety, depression, eating issues) rather than building up a life worth living. Unless they already had past success in employment, strong social networks, and self-sufficiency, there just wasn't enough time in a year of DBT to get to that. Marsha is a brilliant problem-solver, but this was a problem she wasn't regularly targeting in her clinic.

The third reason is this is a really hard therapeutic problem to solve. A metaphor might help explain. Marsha used to tell a story about DBT as the ladder out of hell (this story precedes the house of DBT—similar but more visceral). DBT clients are in hell, a very deep pit with the bottom covered in hot coals. There is only one way out, an aluminum ladder that is as hot to touch as the coals are at the bottom. The client in constant emotional pain or crisis is lying in the coals on the bottom—excruciatingly painful but not requiring effort or skill. The goal of DBT is to help clients climb onto the ladder and keep climbing without jumping off and ending back at the bottom. Since jumping off (e.g., cutting, getting drunk, attempting suicide, or any other escape from pain) is the only pain-free time, it is very tempting to jump off. But, of course, then you end up on the hot coals and have to climb the ladder again. While this truly is an arduous process for clients, Marsha proposed that, part way up, the walls of the pit have ledges and you can get off the ladder and onto the ledges—for the first time in a long time (possibly ever) a place that's not burning hot and doesn't mean falling back into the pit of hell. The emotional pain and crisis have stopped at last. But here is the big, new challenge: How do you get off the ledge and back onto this super-hot ladder and keep climbing it so you can get out of the pit entirely? And how do you do it without retreating to another ledge or, worst-case scenario, jumping off and ending up on the coals where you have to climb the ladder from the bottom again? This is the challenge of DBT Next Steps. We hope it is validating to both clients and their therapists that we assert this problem is very hard to solve; there is nothing wrong with you if you struggle with it.

The Challenges of Targeting QOL-Interfering Behavior

This introductory section of the manual provides background about the experience of individuals with BPD and emotion regulation difficulties and their pursuit of goals related to employment, strong social networks, and self-sufficiency. It provides perspective on why DBT Next Steps, based on DBT-ACES, is needed and why it can be just as intensive a treatment as Standard DBT (SDBT). The bulk of this book (Parts II and IV) is organized into core principles, strategies, and skills used in DBT-ACES that can be integrated into SDBT as needed by the DBT therapist—what we are calling *DBT Next Steps*. In Part III of this book, we integrate these strategies as they are used in the comprehensive DBT-ACES program and include useful logistical steps that make the comprehensive program successful.

As the DBT clinician targets QOL-interfering behavior, they must consider the range of values and aspirations of the client and identify actionable steps to move them toward living a meaningful and fulfilling life. QOL-interfering targets could include decreasing particular behaviors, such as reducing addictive behaviors, interpersonal conflicts, or a pattern of ending commitments prematurely, and so forth. However, QOL targets often involve increasing a set of new behaviors and generalizing them to the client's environment. QOL goals related to employment, for example, involve the client engaging in a range of new actions to approach job listings, attend interviews, and communicate with hiring managers effectively, and the like. Once a job is accepted, clients are then expected to demonstrate a range of behaviors needed to succeed, such as managing time effectively, being easy to work with or around others who aren't, or completing a shift even while experiencing intense urges to leave early.

For the client with chronic emotion dysregulation difficulties, this process poses unique challenges. Employment is a struggle, particularly if the individual has never had a stable work history before. Yet, despite the many challenges, there are many for whom employment is an important life goal. A qualitative study examining client goals for recovery found that 50% of the sample of clients with BPD identified the importance of practical achievements and employment as part of their recovery, and that making progress in pursuing career goals would lead to an increased sense of competence (Katsakou et al., 2012). These findings are supported by other qualitative studies of individuals with BPD who report a strong desire to work (Cunningham et al., 2004).

Psychiatric disability and financial dependency have a range of forms. The state and federal government have designations of disability that indicate an inability to work to make enough to live on (albeit in poverty), and most include mental and psychiatric disorders as the causes of such disability (Department of Social Services, Australian Government, n.d.; Government of Canada, 2015; Social Security Administration, n.d.). Employers often have a similar—although generally short-term—disability designation. Alternatively, there are unofficial versions of disability where family, partners, friends, and religious or other organizations financially support individuals whose psychiatric problems interfere with their ability to work. Individuals who are financially dependent on such informal resources have similar challenges as individuals on psychiatric disability in the community behavioral health system—both "profiles" of financial dependency often have powerful environmental disincentives to working and skills deficits in the ability to find and maintain a job. In all cases, the individual is in a position of dependency—unable to make choices without justification and permission from those funding them—and is more often than not living in poverty or at least way below the socioeconomic standing of their family and friends. In DBT Next Steps, all of these situations are considered a disability, and a psychiatric disability if they are primarily a result of mental or emotional problems.

While there are similarities in how these problems are conceptualized from a DBT Next Steps framework, there are important sociocultural differences among individuals who either receive psychiatric disability or are financially dependent on their family. The process of navigating job prospects and educational opportunities can be quite different. An individual on Medicaid/Medicare, growing up in poverty and with multiple generational exposure to community violence, will encounter numerous hardships navigating employment opportunities compared to an individual labeled "failure to launch" who is dependent on the available financial support from a family with the means to provide it. These two profiles of financial dependency are further illustrated in Chapter 3 with two case examples of clients progressing through SDBT and completing DBT-ACES treatment.

Clients might encounter other challenges when the expectations of their job role are in contrast to their cultural identifications. Thus, a client's work and self-sufficiency needs must be addressed in the context of their cultural background. Bolden et al. (2020) highlighted cultural dialectics in the process of implementing DBT-ACES for multicultural clients (re)entering the workforce. Cultural dialectics refers to a dialectical dilemma in which a client struggles to adhere to a value or norm associated with their culture and the tension of a divergent or opposing value. Clients may not feel comfortable talking freely with their clinician about valuing roles related to multicultural identity as they fear being judged as being counter-mainstream culture or having values that run counter to those of the clinician. The clinician must do an individualized assessment of how the client sees themself in the context of their cultural identifications, taking into account the client's potential discomfort discussing conflicting roles. We will highlight these cultural dialectics with examples throughout this book.

It can be difficult to figure out how to target at the QOL level and clinicians often don't know where to start. This is particularly the case with goals related to school or work or social achievements like a successful best friendship or romantic relationship where the goals seem unattainable to the clinician, let alone the client. The clinician's skepticism or trepidation to move toward seemingly unattainable goals will inevitably influence the client's view about whether their own goals are attainable. This transaction can leave both feeling hesitant to approach life worth living goal-focused activities. Clinicians will sometimes prioritize trauma interventions versus building a stronger base of independence or a stronger social network that would maximize success with exposure strategies. Clinicians also sometimes focus on targets that might not lead to the biggest and most substantive step toward life worth living goals. Perhaps the goals themselves are vague or lack behavioral specificity, whereupon setting specific Action Steps becomes a challenge. For example, the life worth living goal "Feeling better about myself" lacks precision. "Being a highly respected worker who regularly feels competence and confidence while contributing to a sales team" provides more clarity and specificity about an employment goal. Note that this example contains specific activities, and the emotions or experiences prompted by the activities, which can make for a clear, precise, and compelling life worth living goal. Another common challenge is that even when the school or work goal is clear and attainable, clients may engage in a range of avoidance behaviors, leaving clinicians at a loss for how to push forward despite numerous attempts to assess and problem-solve. The client's goals are clear, yet as the weeks turn into months, minimal action is taken to approach them. Finding a path forward through numerous approach–avoid roadblocks can be defeating for clinicians. Their clients remain stuck, and because clients are not reaching substantive life goals, there's a lack of reinforcers for both the client and the clinician.

Why (or Why Not) DBT Next Steps?

The step between the current state and a life worth living often requires a trial by fire—that is, going through something distinctly difficult, like finding a job, applying for school, dating, or joining groups or activities in search of close friends—something that is both harder than what they are doing now and much harder than where the client is trying to get to (i.e., it is much harder to look for work than to work, harder to date than be in a relationship, harder to find friends than to have friends). For the DBT client who has moved beyond crisis behaviors, yet hasn't made progress toward their life worth living goals, depression, anxiety, shame, and suffering in quiet desperation are likely to set in. Suicidal thinking can and has returned for many of our clients. TIBs may arise as clients have hopeless thoughts about their lack of progress. Then the focus goes back to SDBT top targets—ironically, a comfortable place for many DBT therapists—and thus DBT can drag on yet not end as the therapist becomes re-engaged around higher targets.

This side of the dialectic makes it urgent and critical that DBT therapists take their clients through the Next Steps to their life worth living goals. In most DBT research, DBT had to stop at 1 year because that was the research design, not because DBT had done all it could do. If you want DBT to do all it can do, to fulfill the promise of the life worth living goals, you have to get the client through the Next Steps. This book offers key skills and strategies to do this: a roadmap for building self-sufficiency, seeking out new responsibilities and excelling at them, and putting client's skills to the test. This approach to DBT QOL-interfering behaviors that block a life worth living offers new skills, specific QOL targets, a series of graduated contingencies, and exposure strategies that all help clients move forward.

DBT Next Steps helps clients to hold the dialectic that on the one hand, they may have a history of out-of-control behaviors that can appear in many domains of their life and, on the other hand, the frustrations that clients experience day-to-day as they move toward working and self-sufficiency are largely understandable, experienced by most people, and are manageable by developing skills and resilience. DBT Next Steps seeks a synthesis of both validating and overcoming emotion dysregulation problems, while helping clients see how much they share with other unemployed people who have not struggled with emotional problems, with other people faced with the challenge of building something new, with jumping out of the nest without a net and learning to fly. The synthesis is not in ignoring emotional problems or the challenges that accompany them; instead, it is to challenge oneself to accept life's difficulties, accept help and support, and keep taking the next step forward (Comtois et al., 2020). The client has already achieved a lot—they got off the hot coals and climbed the ladder and got to a ledge, drawing from the previous metaphor. We have to help the client to get off the ledge, to get back on the hot ladder, and to get out of the pit of hell.

Yet, of course, there is another side of the dialectic. If the client has life worth living goals of working, getting a degree, moving out on their own, being self-sufficient, having a network of good friends, yet after substantial targeting and trying multiple DBT strategies, they aren't taking these Next Steps, then the clinician and client should consider reasons "why not."

There are clients for whom a year of SDBT has brought about progress toward these goals. If there are clear progress and confidence that the momentum can be sustained even after DBT therapy is over, it's questionable whether the Next Steps need to be taken within psychotherapy. It could well be that therapy has achieved its mission and the client can take it from here. For many clients who have experienced their life worth living goals in the past, now that they have skills and are stable, they are able to jump right back in. We see this a lot for clients with "later-in-life" onset of emotional dysregulation or BPD following a major life change (e.g., divorce, empty nest, loss of a parent, move to a new city, or loss of a long-term job). Once they have behavioral control back, they have the experience and self-efficacy to take the Next Steps and often do so during SDBT. These are often the cases where it feels like DBT is doing the work by itself with little input from the therapist. Trauma is also a source of emotional pain and chronic crisis. These are the clients for whom moving from DBT into a formal trauma exposure protocol works wonders. Once treated, they re-engage with what they have been avoiding and rebuild their life worth living on their own.

Another reason "why not" to take Next Steps is that the person really wants to retire, even if it is from a career as a mental health client. Some people with chronic emotional or psychiatric illness into their fifties and sixties finally find DBT and achieve a level of functioning they haven't had in years. But for them, the time to achieve vocationally and to take risks to be self-sufficient feels in the past or requires a level of energy and engagement they don't have. Sometimes this is because getting through SDBT was really tough and their top targets were established over many years and were very hard to unravel and change. Other times they also have medical or chronic pain conditions that make life a challenge beyond emotional problems. Essentially, the ledge in the pit of hell feels OK and the urgency isn't there to get back onto that hot ladder.

You might be thinking that means their life worth living goals have or should change to something they want to achieve. We think that, too. If so, perhaps there are different Next Steps—reconnection with family, finding a support system in their church or their town, or pursuing a hobby or personal project they value. Some of these are amenable to the DBT Next Steps skills and strategies. Sometimes, it is more a question of finding sufficient support to have security and safety or finding meaning in life. Other therapy models might be more successful and less effortful than DBT.

Examining the research highlights the "why not" reasons. We found half or fewer of our SDBT clients continue to DBT-ACES. Other SDBT clients did not need it because they were already taking the Next Steps, had dropped out of SDBT, did not stabilize during SDBT, or decided that getting off of disability and returning to work or school was not their priority (Comtois et al., 2010, 2020).

In summary, we suggest that the primary question is not "Why pursue DBT Next Steps?," but instead, "Why would you *not* pursue DBT Next Steps?" If the answer is emotional avoidance then we know the answer. Emotional avoidance is not a reason to do much of anything. If the answer is the therapist doesn't know what to do to target this kind of avoidance or how to use exposure and contingency management to promote life worth living goals, or the client doesn't have the skills they need—then the answer lies in this book.

Core Concepts: Psychiatric Disability and Normative Functioning

Individuals with BPD or emotion dysregulation have unique challenges for building financial self-sufficiency. Psychiatric disability refers to the inability to earn sufficient income to meet basic needs. Individuals with psychiatric disability are often engaged in mental health services with the hope of ameliorating disability—these services range from pharmacotherapy alone to long-term individual psychotherapy to community mental health, partial hospital, intensive outpatient, clubhouse, or other intensive services. If not supported by family wealth, these individuals are generally embedded in a range of social services beyond mental health including disability income from employers or the state, public insurance programs, public housing, food stamps, and other programs supporting social welfare. Unfortunately, from a behavioral point of view, many of these programs are withdrawn or include disincentives for engaging in normative behaviors, particularly paid employment. Families and employers likewise can withdraw financial support when the disabled individual gets a job or returns to work or otherwise shows improvement. Our goal in DBT Next Steps is to find a dialectical synthesis by focusing on self-sufficiency and school or employment as key steps toward recovery and normative functioning while buffering the loss of resources that comes with making such a change.

We define "normative functioning" as "acting as if you don't have emotional problems around others who are acting as if they don't have emotional problems." This applies to work, school, social contacts, and community living (e.g., dealing with the bank, medical providers, insurance agents and government officials, washing the dishes, paying the bills). Generally, the others don't have significant emotional problems, and the key issue is that the setting is "normative" if it is not defined by its members' emotional problems or psychiatric illness (e.g., not a community mental health center, sheltered workshop, clubhouse). We have found that individuals with BPD are very sensitive to the expectations of those around them and that they have more success in environments where the focus is off their emotional and psychiatric problems. Many of our clients have found it easier to not disclose their emotional problems to members of these new settings and communities. When the community only expects normative behavior, it appears to help clients to produce it.

Normative Productivity is referred to as both a broader concept and a behavioral contingency woven into DBT Next Steps. The goal of the Normative Productive Activities requirement is to increase exposure to social settings and expand opportunities to act skillfully, while working to decrease depression and anxiety that are often associated with social isolation, unstructured time, and limited demands outside of the home. The "three S's" of Normative Productivity focus on the quality of the activities that are chosen to ensure that they are (1) Structured, (2) Scheduled, and (3) Social. Normative Productive Activities (or the less formal name, "Getting Active") are expected to occur in SDBT ahead of DBT Next Steps so that there is already behavioral activation and exposure in place, which the therapist and client can shape toward approaching school or work goals. A metaphor here is that it's easier to climb the mountain if you already have hiking shoes that are broken in and have scaled a few foothills first. Normative Productivity offers the opportunity to increase behavioral activation and practice being skillful in settings that are structured, scheduled, and social. Once these foothills are climbed, then the client will more easily be able to increase the incline and do the more difficult climbing of approaching work, school, and other life worth living goals.

Once a client can do Normative Productive Activities, the therapist pursuing Next Steps can build in one or both graduated contingencies in DBT Next Steps: Career Activities and Work as Therapy. Career Activities focus on the steps needed for living-wage employment in a desired career by building in activities that move the client forward along their career path. Work as Therapy provides exposure to work environments and demands. In addition to habituating to the emotions associated with working, the client gains work experience where they are effective, and this facilitates their independence from psychiatric disability programs, the social service system, and family or friends' financial support as the client gradually increases their work hours or gets raises and promotions.

To move past avoidance and on to life worth living goals, our aspiration is that the skills the clients have learned and the environmental contingencies clients have created for themselves provide sufficient momentum so it is almost inevitable that they will achieve their employment, social, and independence goals (without having to stay in DBT for the entire journey). Being able to move forward in the face of the many disincentives for achieving financial independence is truly what is called for to escape the many ways that the system and individuals in one's environment inadvertently hold clients back. If the client needs the environment to be sufficiently hospitable to achieve success, the client will likely be blocked almost immediately in their process to return to work and shift their pattern of dependency on others. That is why DBT-ACES stands for Accepting the Challenges of Employment and Self-Sufficiency: Because it is a challenge that cannot be avoided, it must be accepted and overcome. Chapter 7 provides more details of these graduated contingencies that are built into DBT Next Steps to help clients cross the divide between the desire to work and actually being employed.

Overview of DBT Next Steps and the Comprehensive DBT-ACES Program

The comprehensive DBT-ACES program is an expansion and adaptation of SDBT designed to meet the needs of individuals with emotion dysregulation problems who are psychiatrically disabled or financially dependent on others. As described earlier, DBT-ACES was developed in response to the heartbreak we experienced as a consultation team when deeply entrenched and complex clients didn't achieve the lives they wanted after SDBT treatment. DBT-ACES created the structure and contingencies our psychiatrically disabled clients needed to make significant progress and gain momentum toward their life worth living goals. Piloting DBT-ACES didn't have positive effects only on our clients (Comtois et al., 2010), it also had positive effects on our consultation team. Clinician burnout was reduced simply by hearing from our clients who graduated from DBT-ACES, telling us of their productive, meaningful, or at least above-average lives with jobs they were excited about, or their connection to friends, family, and community.

Program evaluations of DBT-ACES have demonstrated suicide-related outcomes comparable to those of clinical trials as well as promising findings for increasing school and work activities and meaningful cost benefits. The results of a feasibility trial found that clients in DBT-ACES were three times more likely to be working or in school and five times more likely to be working 20 hours a week or more in the year of DBT-ACES than their SDBT year (Comtois et al., 2010). A three-site evaluation including programs in Germany and California has replicated and exceeded these pre–post results and included a cost–benefit analysis yielding substantial savings (Carmel et al., 2021; Comtois et al., 2020). While the majority of the over $17,000 per DBT-ACES client cost-offset compared to the year prior to SDBT was primarily driven by the decrease in inpatient care, evidence of significant school and workplace benefits was also observed in SDBT and particularly in DBT-ACES compared to the year prior to SDBT (Comtois et al., 2020). In addition to these effectiveness studies, several articles have been published on the clinical application of DBT-ACES. These articles include a case study of the progression from SDBT through DBT-ACES (Comtois et al., 2020), considerations for integrating DBT-ACES components into CBT (Carmel & Comtois, 2023), and examining cultural dialectics while providing DBT-ACES in multicultural community mental health settings (Bolden et al., 2020).

In this book, we do not expect that the majority of therapists and DBT programs will want to implement the comprehensive DBT-ACES program as designed. Many programs that are considering implementing in any capacity might consider a synthesis of integrating only certain strategies while tracking clinical outcomes and acceptability among clinical staff. This will provide the data needed to guide decisions to expand to other strategies or skills. A program might see the value of integrating certain components of DBT-ACES for patients who have moved from overtly out-of-control behaviors to avoidance of behaviors they need to increase. The DBT Next Steps strategies described in Part II of this book might be implemented as a whole for clients as they reach this stage of treatment, or implemented individually, strategy by strategy. In such a circumstance, individual therapist–client dyads pick up more and more Next Steps approaches, and a DBT Next Steps skills group can be available for clients, but, unlike DBT-ACES, it is not treated as a separate program requiring an explicit decision to enter through a formal pretreatment process and doesn't have an explicit time limit or other formal structure. In this way, DBT Next Steps can be incorporated like other evidence-based modalities in DBT.

Therefore, the bulk of this book (Parts II and IV) is organized into core principles, strategies, and skills used in DBT-ACES that can be integrated into SDBT as needed by the DBT therapist—what we are calling DBT Next Steps. In Part III of this book, we integrate these strategies back into the comprehensive DBT-ACES program and include useful logistical steps that make the comprehensive program successful (see Chapters 11 and 12). Then in Chapter 13, we consider the pros and cons of incorporating some or all components of DBT Next Steps within SDBT or implementing all of the components as a comprehensive DBT-ACES program. In Part IV of this book, we include all of the teaching notes and lesson plans for the DBT Next Steps skills curriculum. These teaching notes correspond with the companion volume to this text, *DBT Next Steps Skills Handouts*, which features all of the skills-training handouts and assignments for clients.

CHAPTER 2

Structural Differences between Standard DBT and DBT Next Steps

The goal of the Next Steps is to keep the clients moving as they come out of Stage 1 behavioral dyscontrol (i.e., moving farther from their life worth living goals) to Stage "1a," where avoidance or lack of skill prevents them from moving toward their life worth living goals, as shown in Figure 2.1.

The principle of DBT Next Steps across the board is that to move from tearing their life down to building it up, clients must become more competent in skills emphasizing self-sufficiency, be exposed to feared cues, and create strong environmental contingencies that reinforce taking action toward their goals as well as emotional and financial independence. Yet navigating this process will require the DBT therapist to address systemic hardships and other aspects of multicultural identity that might pose critical challenges for the individual as they pursue school, work, a strong social network, and self-sufficiency goals. The challenges experienced by the clients might be unknown or hidden to the therapist who possesses more privilege. Some DBT therapists treating the client labeled as "failure to launch" might employ a more

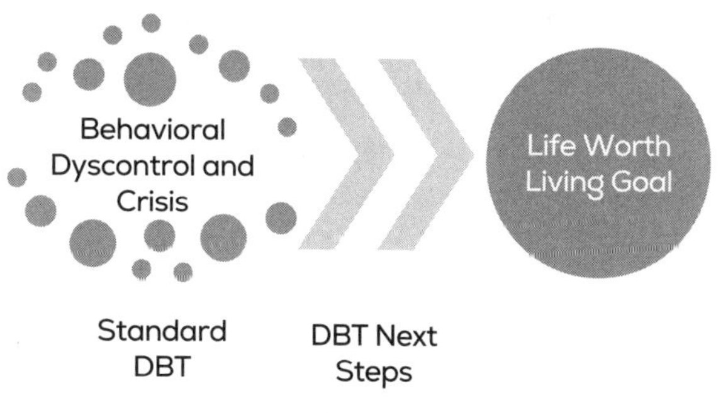

FIGURE 2.1. Progression out of Stage 1 to Stage 1a.

nuanced assessment of the disincentives for working and consider environmental reinforcement of emotion dysregulation or dependency behavior. They might consider, for example, that the client exists within invalidating environments where other family members thrive and succeed and the client doesn't; where there is an oversimplification of the ease of developing and excelling in one's career.

On the flip side, for those living on a lower income or in more communal cultures, self-sufficiency needs to be considered in context. Counting on others for financial, housing, transportation, child care, and other resources may not only be expected but also valued, with the goal being interdependence. This is consistent with the Principle of Interrelatedness and Wholeness articulated by Linehan (1993) in the core text of DBT. In this spirit, a dialectical look at self-sufficiency highlights that one cannot (and probably should not) strive for full independence—not needing anyone else to get along. This standard is perfectionistic and inconsistent with many cultures and community values. On the other hand, we can observe many cases of dependency that are problematic across cultures and contexts—this is often seen in the secondary target of active passivity and when family or friends offer opportunities or supports and the client's avoidance prevents them from taking action. This leaves both the client and their community—as well as their therapist—frustrated and stuck. DBT Next Steps uses the term "self-sufficiency" with this dialectic in mind: What does the client need to be able to do for themself to be effective in and a valued member of their community or subculture?

DBT Next Steps achieves this through targeted skills training with a new skills curriculum as well as unique contingency management and *in vivo* exposure-based strategies that function to initiate and maintain self-sufficiency and achieve goals—as well as to proactively structure one's environment to facilitate these behaviors. The following section provides a reminder of SDBT targets, strategies, and functions before illustrating the adapted approach of DBT Next Steps to address these challenges.

Summary of SDBT

DBT is defined by its philosophical base (dialectics), treatment strategies, and treatment targets. The term "dialectical" is meant to convey both the multiple tensions that co-occur in therapy with emotionally dysregulated clients as well as the emphasis in DBT of enhancing dialectical thinking patterns to replace rigid, dichotomous thinking (Linehan, 1993). The overriding dialectic is the acceptance of clients as they are within the context of helping them change. DBT requires that each therapist working with the client balance the use of strategies, from the rapid juxtaposition of change and acceptance foci to the use of both irreverent and warmly responsive communication styles. Strategy changes in DBT are required to maintain therapeutic progress in the face of a client who, at various moments, may oscillate between suicidal crises, rigid refusal to collaborate, rapid emotional escalation, and collaborative effort.

SDBT Treatment Targets

DBT treatment targets for suicidal clients are organized in a hierarchy, with the top priority being life-threatening behaviors including suicidal behaviors, nonsuicidal self-injury, and violence toward others. The second target is TIB, which includes clients' nonattendance, noncompliance, and noncollaborative behaviors or therapists being out of balance in their use of DBT strategies or being disrespectful. The third target is QOL-interfering behaviors including psychiatric disorders, substance abuse, unemployment, interpersonal conflicts, and so forth. The fourth target is to increase the client's mastery of DBT skills, and the fifth and final target focus is on any other client goals.

SDBT Strategies

DBT treatment strategies are divided into five sets: (1) dialectical strategies; (2) core strategies (validation and problem solving), including standard CBT procedures (behavioral assessment, didactic strategies, orienting to treatment rationale, contingency management, skills training, exposure, and cognitive modification strategies); (3) communication strategies (irreverent and reciprocal communication styles); (4) case management strategies (consultation to the client, environmental intervention, consultation to the therapists); and (5) structural strategies (targeting within sessions, starting and ending therapy). There are also a number of specific behavioral treatment protocols covering how to respond to suicidal behaviors and other crises states, TIBs and compliance issues, relationship problems and breakdowns, as well as ancillary treatment issues, including medication management.

SDBT Functions

SDBT serves five functions: (1) increasing behavioral capabilities; (2) improving motivation for more skillful responding, by modifying inhibitions and reinforcement contingencies; (3) assuring that treatment gains generalize to the natural environment; (4) structuring the treatment environment so that it reinforces functional rather than dysfunctional behaviors; and (5) enhancing therapist capabilities and motivation to treat clients effectively.

SDBT Modes of Treatment Delivery

These functions are divided among four modes of service delivery, each described in detail below.

1. **Weekly individual psychotherapy** (1 hour/week) functions primarily to improve client's motivation to reduce dysfunctional behaviors and replace them with functional and effective behaviors. It is designed to provide individualized behavioral assessment, treatment planning, and change strategies aimed at helping clients inhibit maladaptive behaviors and instead use behavioral skills, even if newly learned, in problematic situations. Session agendas are determined by treatment targets. If the client is at risk for imminent suicidal behavior or self-injury, crisis intervention takes priority. If maladaptive behaviors in the first three DBT target areas have occurred since the previous sessions (as indicated by reviewing the weekly Diary Card) or occur during the session, then those behaviors are the focus of the session. Generally, this involves an intensive analysis of the specific problem behavior in question (vulnerability and contextual factors, prompting events, behavioral links up to the problem behavior, consequences), and in-session interventions and out-of-session homework focus on what is needed

for the client to avoid their problematic response in the future. If no problems in these areas have arisen, then problems or issues the client wants to work on determine the focus of the session. The primary focus is on analyzing and changing associations and contingencies to inhibit dysfunctional behaviors, particularly those associated with suicidality and BPD criteria, and to shape alternative skillful responses. Environmental intervention (e.g., interacting with other professionals or friends and family to manage services or circumstances for the client) occurs only when the immediate safety of the client outweighs the loss of opportunity for shaping new client behaviors (by teaching clients how to handle the problem themselves) or when the social power of the client is insufficient to effect necessary change (e.g., a letter from a clinician is required to get public housing).

2. **Group skills training** (2.5 hours/week) functions to enhance the acquisition of new behavioral skills. It is didactically focused and emphasizes modeling, instructions, structured behavioral rehearsal exercises, feedback, and assignments to practice new skills. In contrast to individual therapy, the session agenda is determined by the skills to be taught, rather than by maladaptive behaviors of the clients. Assignments are reviewed during the first half of the session and new material (with handouts) is taught during the second half. The structured skills manual gives session-by-session guidelines for content and format (Linehan, 2025b). There are four group skill modules targeting (a) mindfulness, (b) interpersonal effectiveness, (c) emotion regulation, and (d) distress tolerance skills. The latter three modules are given once over the course of 6 months, and mindfulness is taught for 2 weeks before each module. Problems not specifically related to skills, such as suicide threats or complex difficulties applying skills to individual situations, are referred to the individual therapist. In SDBT, the skills trainer meets with the individual DBT therapist in weekly team consultation.

3. **Out-of-session coaching** (as needed within the therapist's limits)—usually by phone but increasingly by text or other messaging platforms—functions to enhance the strength and generalization of learning to the client's everyday environment. Brief telephone contact between sessions, within the personal limits of each individual therapist and their client, is used for (a) problem solving and coaching in generalization of skills, (b) crisis intervention, (c) reinforcement of effective behavior, and (d) relationship repair.

4. **Therapists' team consultation** (weekly) functions to enhance and maintain therapists' motivation and skill. All therapists attend a structured weekly meeting to assist each other in the implementation of the treatment. The goal is dialectical—to help therapists to accept themselves, each other, and the clients and to mobilize themselves, each other, and the clients to change.

DBT Next Steps Modes of Treatment Delivery

DBT Next Steps is structurally and fundamentally DBT. It has the same functions as DBT and uses all the principles, assumptions, agreements, and treatment strategies. The balance of acceptance-based and change-based strategies is done in the effort to help clients accept the challenges of increasing self-sufficiency and taking action toward life worth living goals while providing the tools necessary to do so. Secondary targets in DBT Next Steps are identical to secondary targets in SDBT. The following sections outline each treatment mode, highlight changes, and address pitfalls that can arise when doing DBT Next Steps.

Individual DBT

Individual therapy is fundamentally identical to individual therapy in SDBT. As in SDBT, the weekly individual therapy sessions are the mode around which all other treatment modes revolve. The individual therapist is responsible for identifying client goals, behavioral assessment, and implementing the core validation, problem-solving, and dialectical strategies, and for applying the primary contingency, skills training, exposure and cognitive modification change procedures, and all other DBT strategies.

The differences in DBT Next Steps individual sessions stem from the higher functioning and enhanced skillfulness of the clients, which are critical to reinforce. There is relatively more emphasis on cueing client's effective behavior than blocking dysfunctional behavior or teaching new behavior. Also, though the primary SDBT targets of (1) life-threatening behavior, (2) TIB, and (3) dangerous and out-of-control QOL-interfering behaviors remain as primary targets and are monitored each week, they are expected to be infrequent so rarely take up individual session time. Instead, the targeting is focused on the QOL-interfering behaviors characterized by avoidance—situations where the client is not taking action or building something new. Such behaviors lend themselves to a full range of exposure strategies and manualized behavioral treatments for other psychiatric disorders (e.g., activation treatment for depression or CBT for social phobia), and it is more likely that a client can see such therapy protocols through to the end than is typical with beginning SDBT clients. Thus, a major difference is that the therapist exercises more cueing strategies than skills-training strategies, thereby relying more on the client to manage the agenda and the basic steps of the session, and to identify and apply appropriate skills.

Two main pitfalls when moving from targeting behavioral dyscontrol to targeting avoidance of self-sufficiency, employment, and the like in individual sessions are (1) escalation of self-harm, crisis-generating, or therapy-interfering behaviors and (2) loss of client or therapist motivation (urgency) prior to reaching life worth living goal milestones.

When focusing on Next Steps in individual sessions, any escalation of self-harm, crisis-generating, or therapy-interfering behavior requires the same set of acceptance and change strategies on the part of the therapist as in SDBT. Often such an escalation occurs when goals have been set too high; however, such escalation can also function as avoidance for the client. Such "bursts" of previous dysfunctional behavior are common in SDBT and can be more demoralizing to the client and therapist when moving on to DBT Next Steps. However, the principles for responding are identical in the two treatments and comparable to those of DBT trauma interventions such as the DBT Prolonged Exposure protocol (DBT PE; Carmel et al., 2016).

During DBT Next Steps individual sessions, the client or therapist may experience reduced motivation, resulting in an inclination to settle for less than the original goals. While this sense of complacency is certainly understandable, it is exactly the opposite of what is needed. When this happens to the therapist, the same disciplined self-monitoring and consultation team intervention is required as in SDBT. Similarly, when this occurs in the client, the therapist applies the same validation, commitment, dialectical and contingency highlighting, and management strategies as in SDBT.

Group Skills Training

The DBT Next Steps skills-training six-module curriculum is taught in one 2-hour group per week. Each of the Next Steps modules lasts 1 month, so completing the entire curriculum of six modules takes 6 months. These skills build on SDBT skills but are distinct. DBT Next Steps skills handouts and assignments can be found in our companion book for clients, *DBT Next Steps Skills Handouts,* and detailed lesson plans for skills group leaders can be found in Part IV of this volume. The same clinical and didactic strategies are used in SDBT and Next Steps groups. Similar to SDBT skills modules, the Next Steps skills modules include both acceptance-oriented and change-oriented skills.

Out-of-Session Coaching

Out-of-session coaching via telephone, text, or other messaging platforms is provided as in SDBT, except the focus is on coaching self-sufficiency as opposed to generating solutions for the clients. In SDBT, out-of-session coaching in which the client contacts the therapist for *in vivo* coaching can be utilized as both a crisis management intervention and an opportunity to focus on cueing and reinforcing early skill acquisition as well as generalization. In DBT Next Steps, telephone consultations differ in that they emphasize consultation-to-patient strategies aimed primarily at skills generalization, although there is also ample opportunity to cue and reinforce early acquisition of DBT Next Steps skills. There is less need for the crisis management function as clients should already have distress tolerance solidly in their skills repertoire.

The pitfalls of coaching when working on Next Steps are that (1) coaching may be underutilized due to its association in SDBT with crisis behavior, and (2) coaching can interfere with "self-sufficiency" targets by inadvertently reinforcing reliance on cueing from the therapist.

The association with "crisis management" in SDBT treatment makes it a challenge for clients and clinicians to adapt to a more developmentally appropriate use of out-of-session coaching. For clinicians, this is dealt with in a consultation team, with regular reminders to assess the utility of coaching sessions and any possible unwitting reinforcement of avoidance behavior on the part of the client. When focused on DBT Next Steps, clinicians also use coaching as a vehicle for clients to report their use of skills and effective behavior, rather than reaching out only when they need help. Reinforcement of adaptive behavior is extremely important as clients overcome their anxiety and shame, and re-approach the workforce, social community, and so forth. It is typical to have planned contact after clients take action for themselves, or to have a general expectation of update messages to which the therapist can send congratulatory memes or emojis. Similar to contingency management in addiction treatment, these communications provide extra reinforcement during the period when natural reinforcements are not present and can be tapered once natural reinforcers begin to surface. There are many more reinforcers to working or attending school versus filling out applications, being in relationships versus dating or finding friends, and being settled in one's own place versus saving up and moving. For clients, getting oriented to the differences in how telephone coaching is used is a key part of becoming oriented to DBT Next Steps. The clinician must communicate the challenges of adapting, while holding to the rationale of adapting—that these changes promote more self-generated skills practice so that clients are able to reach their life worth living goals. Once the client has overcome the initial hurdles and is working, in school, living on their own, and the like, coaching as an outside support can be tapered prior to the end of treatment.

Therapist Consultation Team

As in SDBT, the weekly consultation team meetings include all individual and group therapists and serve to assure treatment fidelity by providing therapists with skills, support, and re-moralization as they implement the treatment strategies. The same elements are required for DBT consultation to be effective for Next Steps as well as for treating behavioral dyscontrol. All therapists must make and keep the supervision/consultation agreements, cheerlead other therapists, maintain a balance of acceptance and change strategies, and maintain the integrity of the "team" as an active agent in the therapy. In both treatments, the consultation team is also where the team devises and authorizes the application of specific contingencies, such as individually tailored changes in behavioral expectations, requirements for collateral substance abuse treatment when it is necessary, or therapy suspensions (a.k.a. vacations).

The main pitfall of consultation team meetings for clinicians working with DBT Next Steps clients is that it is more challenging to observe and review incremental improvements in QOL-interfering behaviors, like the absence or avoidance of something, than behavioral dyscontrol (e.g., not submitting job applications vs. bingeing and purging). This can be addressed by giving a block of consultation team time each quarter (maybe 30–45 minutes depending on how many clients are working in DBT Next Steps) to focus on the current clients pursuing Next Steps and whether the individual therapists are targeting effectively. In our team, we have tied this to the Recovery Goals (discussed in Chapter 4), and we have found it helpful to tie these team discussions to when the clients conduct a reassessment of the Recovery Goals in their skills-training group (see the Self-Assessment of Recovery Goals form in *DBT Next Steps Skills Handouts*). Looking at the client's assessment of themself, the therapist can see how their targeting is doing compared to the client's view. The team can discuss changes that need to be made or do "therapy for the therapist" if the therapist knows what to do and isn't doing it.

DBT Next Steps Strategies

DBT integrates a range of treatment strategies that balance acceptance with change. The DBT therapist targeting a client's negative self-talk and self-invalidation, for example, might use acceptance-based strategies such as Mindfulness of Current Thoughts to coach the client to observe the thought arising and notice it passing. On the other hand, they might just as easily use change-based approaches such as Checking the Facts or highlighting the consequences of getting stuck in self-invalidating thoughts and consider alternative ways to respond.

There are four primary change procedures to draw from in SDBT: exposure strategies, contingency management, cognitive modification, and behavioral skills training. Just as in SDBT, DBT Next Steps uses change procedures to increase learning in all relevant contexts where new behaviors are needed. For example, a client might be coached to validate their therapist's perspective even though they adamantly disagree with it. While there might be more validation seen in session, what's ultimately needed for the client to thrive is the ability to generalize perspective taking and find validity in a vastly different point of view from their partner, teacher, or manager in a work setting. While change procedures are used by all SDBT therapists, DBT Next Steps emphasizes them in particular ways that block avoidance and reinforce courageous new behaviors required for the client's life worth living.

In order to accomplish this, the therapist keeps an eye out for the deficits or problems that arise in the client's life. What is needed in their job role and what are they demonstrating in session or other contexts? As in SDBT, the appropriate change procedure is selected to address the problem at hand. Consider the contexts where new behaviors are required in order for the client to meet their goals. Perhaps unwarranted shame or fear limits full participation or attendance. In this case, exposure might be the way to go. Are effective behaviors such as submitting job applications getting followed by neutral or punishing responses from others in their life, such as a parent questioning the client's readiness to pull it off? Contingency management is worth exploring. Consider if the client has a lack of awareness of the consequences following their avoidance behavior. Cognitive modification might be needed. Or does the client lack skills to manage time, build a sufficient sense of community to create a work/life balance, or get stuck in the rut of perfectionism? Then skills training addressing these specific skills deficits will be key to success.

In summary, the targets and balance of strategies in DBT for building a new life may be different than SDBT for behavioral dyscontrol, but the treatment is still fundamentally DBT. One key difference is the ability to see the avoidance behavior clearly and understand the internal and external contingencies that make sense of the client's avoidance behavior. The other is the strategic use of DBT principles and strategies to overcome this avoidance. To further illustrate these ideas, two case examples are presented in the next chapter and continue throughout this book.

CHAPTER 3

Case Examples

Application of DBT Next Steps in Two Different Cases of Disability

The following two case examples illustrate the progression through SDBT and the process of applying and completing a DBT Next Steps program, with the details changed to protect against identification.

Case Example: Janet

This case demonstrates the application of DBT Next Steps in the treatment of a chronically suicidal client receiving Medicaid (i.e., public health insurance for disability) who had stabilized while in SDBT at a community mental health clinic, and who was motivated to enter the comprehensive DBT-ACES program. The background of the case is presented, followed by a description of individual and group treatment, including how the graduated contingencies were used to promote self-sufficiency.

Janet (she/her) is a 45-year-old, biracial (Asian American and White), cisgender, heterosexual, single female who was referred to outpatient DBT at a community mental health center for the management of chronic suicidality and self-harm behavior of cutting. She had been in and out of mental health treatment since she was 16. Despite ongoing psychotherapy and case management, she continued to experience significant symptoms of panic, depression, and post-traumatic stress disorder (PTSD). Janet had been admitted, voluntarily, to an acute psychiatric inpatient unit two times in the previous 3 years following suicide attempts by overdosing on prescription medication. When she began SDBT, she was being supported by a cash allowance of $330 per month from the state for psychiatric disability, on Medicaid, and living in low-income housing.

Janet spent a year in SDBT, which initially focused on commitment to closing the door to self-harm and learning skills to regulate and manage emotions. She responded well to DBT and began experiencing a reduction in ideation and urges to self-harm starting in month 3. When DBT-ACES was first discussed at month 6 of SDBT, Janet thought about suicide "peripherally, rather than focusing on it all the time," and, although she would occasionally have urges to self-harm, she was able to surf the urge rather than act on it.

Throughout her life, Janet had held several jobs. Due to emotion dysregulation and interpersonal skills deficits, the longest she had maintained a job was 10 months at a local donut shop. She had lost jobs for various reasons, including being fired for getting so angry and frustrated with coworkers that she walked out, and depression and low mood that interfered with attendance and timeliness. Janet's life worth living goals were to have a lucrative career, get off disability and be self-sufficient, become more active in her church community, and one day have a partner and a garden, which would allow her to sell veggies at the local farmers' market to supplement her income. However, Janet was not clear what job she wanted to pursue as she had not considered an inspiring career path consistently. Janet would discuss going back to school to get a degree and would be discouraged by her friends and family because of the demands and stress that such a course of action would place on her. Several years prior to her participation in DBT, she had enrolled in a job-training program; however, she eventually "lost interest" and dropped out. When she started in DBT-ACES, she had not worked in 3 years, and each time she considered returning to work, her fear increased and her urges to kill herself would spike. This resulted in her avoiding job opportunities and deciding to "wait to return to work when I am feeling more confident." This idea of waiting until she was more confident and stable was reinforced by the majority of Janet's close family members and friends. Thus, fear and social expectations were functioning to reinforce avoidance of work and school activities.

At the 6-month point of SDBT, Janet's therapist oriented her to DBT-ACES and discussed the possibility of continuing their work together in DBT-ACES after SDBT, with returning to work and finding a career path as the emphases of her treatment. Though Janet was scared, she consulted her Wise Mind and found that this was something she wanted and needed to pursue. As the SDBT year progressed, the therapist continued to target increased participation in social activities and volunteering through the use of the Normative Productivity contingency and building in structured, scheduled, and social weekly Getting Active hours. As of month 8, Janet began assuming more responsibility in her housing environment and attended church activities more frequently, often staying after services to join in discussions and activities with fellow congregants. Janet experienced this increase in activity as a positive development after an initial spike in fear. The majority of her activities were within a community where she felt "safe" and knew most of the other people.

From a behavioral shaping perspective of reinforcing steps toward a desired behavior, this was progress! Janet and her therapist would take time in session to celebrate each success but also acknowledge that in order to build the life she desired, it would require her stepping outside of her housing and faith community and interacting with people with whom she was not as familiar. Given her drive to do DBT-ACES, she began to create a résumé (getting assistance from others as needed), and eventually, she applied for several jobs at local coffee shops. The focus of SDBT at this time was largely on exposure and shaping (reinforcing small steps toward the desired behavior), including looking over examples of résumés, drafting two bullet points of a résumé, then moving toward fuller drafting, all the way to reinforcing the larger steps of contacting people to ask about their willingness to serve as a reference, and then sharing her draft with others to get feedback. Thinking about work and casually looking for jobs online would often prompt shame. When she experienced shame, Janet's typical response was increased self-invalidation, negative self-talk, catastrophizing thinking, suicidal thoughts, social isolation, and believing that she would never be stable enough to work. She would then escape the situation and continue to avoid. Janet and her therapist worked together to gradually expose her to fear-provoking situations and increasing interpersonal skills as her interviews came and went.

Janet submitted her DBT-ACES application in her 10th month of SDBT and started DBT-ACES after graduating from SDBT. After a couple of months, she started a job in an antiques shop. (*Note:* This job met the Work as Therapy requirement although it wasn't aligned with her desired career.) Soon after starting work, she was given the responsibility of opening and closing the business; this prompted additional fear and anxiety for her as these tasks came with more responsibility than she was accustomed to. The feared catastrophe of this responsibility was making an error with managing payment and being fired, or worse, charged. The therapist worked to increase exposure to taking on these tasks and encouraging Janet to take in evidence to support the notion that she was a productive and respected coworker, even if she made errors.

While Janet was meeting her Work as Therapy contingency at the antiques shop, this was not the type of work she wanted to continue as a career. Therefore, she needed to begin considering what to do for her Career Activities. A target of individual therapy was applying skills to throw herself into her current job and, dialectically, to search for a job that better fit her personality and values. Though the client was now employed, she really didn't like her job at all. She experienced ongoing judgment of the people who lived in that neighborhood and formed negative appraisals of her coworkers and customers. Janet also believed that she was being judged by most people she encountered at work and experienced ongoing shame, anger, fear, and guilt. Individual sessions focused on cueing her to increase mindfulness, using opposite action, and tolerating emotions that prompted misery until she was able to problem-solve and land a job that would be a better fit.

In Janet's Career Plan that she created for her DBT-ACES application, she had focused on becoming a dietician or nutritionist; she had an interest in pursuing this goal since speaking with an acquaintance who shared how much he enjoyed working as a registered dietician. The Career Plan outlined Career Development hours that would start in month 4 of DBT-ACES and build throughout the year. The initial proposal on these hours included many hours of independent research to gain information about the field; however, the therapist proposed that rather than "playing it safe" and pursuing career development hours in isolation, online, from the comfort of her own home while "researching," it would be better to set aside these hours for social and interactive activities. To increase commitment to the idea of building more exposure, the therapist highlighted that if Janet were pursuing a highly social career path as a dietician, then treatment would have to focus on building more opportunities to practice interpersonal effectiveness and exposure to these new settings to offer the best preparation and practice for her. Janet then revised her Career Plan to include more social activities and downplay "researching" activities, including forming a "workgroup" of two to three other people recruited online who were interested in pursuing dietician work. She coordinated their weekly meetings to reflect on relevant dietician blogs and review templates for nutrition plans and methods of tracking patients' dietary intake. She also incorporated an hour a week of "shadowing" her dietician friend and a few other dieticians whom she had contacted, by observing them as they analyzed their patients' health status and educated their patients. The activities of these hours fit the spirit of Career Development—seeking out opportunities to stretch limits and increase exposure to new settings—carrying forward the frame of Normative Productivity and the "three S's": structured, scheduled, and social activities.

Janet's Career Plan included taking courses toward a 2-year degree that she would need to be qualified to pursue independent work as a dietician. Janet's plan was to return to school at her local community college; however, in order to do that, she needed to first repay her financial aid debt. The first months of her DBT-ACES group check-ins centered around the steps she needed to take to re-enroll in school and pay off her debt, with the DBT-ACES group therapists reinforcing all adaptive behavior and blocking avoidance. Her DBT-ACES individual sessions focused on exposure to shame and fear, as well as increasing Janet's self-validation, self-acceptance, and compassion. Outside of work contexts, the therapist coached Janet to take steps to form relationships in environments where she didn't identify as someone with a mental health issue, or at the very least, where her communication with others did not focus exclusively on mental health issues. Her therapist collaborated with her to identify other people and events to engage with and did role-plays on how to interact with new people and acquaintances in such a way that she could continue to develop and enhance the friendship with them if she chose. The therapist also coached Janet not to do or say things that might erode her self-respect or jeopardize the relationships. Skills coaching centered around the application of these interpersonal skills to situations where self-respect and the relationship were both relevant, coaching on a new style of interacting that was needed to preserve both.

In order to regulate her interpersonal responses in these new environments, Janet had to work to regulate her emotional responses. Strengthening skills from the Managing Emotions Effectively DBT Next Steps skills module became a focus of individual sessions. Applying these skills helped her to effectively identify the contexts where dysregulation was most likely to occur, and to pinpoint "irritants" and manage her irritability. She also practiced the skills in this module focusing on cognitive restructuring and expanded Progressive Muscle Relaxation procedures to regulate the primary emotional response of fear that would often be followed by a secondary emotional response of anger and create problematic interactions in social settings.

At the time of Janet's graduation after her year in DBT-ACES, she was due to start school the following week, and despite a Wise Mind offer from her therapist to extend therapy for a month to help apply skills to cope with the transition, she declined. Janet's own Wise Mind was insistent that she had the skills and wherewithal to do it on her own, using only her own natural social supports that had changed quite a bit after she worked to observe her limits with family and friends and to apply similar interpersonal skills related to self-respect and enhancing the relationship.

Case Example: Lee

This case demonstrates the application of DBT-ACES in the treatment of a client with significant substance use problems and difficulty functioning across a range of life domains, seen as having a "failure to launch" as part of the referral to SDBT in a private practice. Lee was ambivalent about starting SDBT as well as applying to DBT-ACES; however, his values and goals related to self-sufficiency were clear even if his career goals were not. The background of the case is presented, followed by a description of individual and group treatment, including how the DBT-ACES contingencies were used to promote self-sufficiency.

Lee (he/him) is a 23-year-old White, cisgender, single, gay male referred to outpatient DBT in private practice for the management of substance abuse, self-harm behavior of head banging, attention-deficit/hyperactivity disorder (ADHD), anxiety and depression, and a dependency on family for managing many of his financial, medical, and self-management needs—a pattern that had spanned his adolescence and appeared to intensify during early adulthood. He was described as a "failure to launch" case in the referral paperwork from his psychiatrist. He had been in and out of mental health and substance abuse treatment since he began having anxiety symptoms and substance use problems at age 12. Starting in high school, his gaming and social media use spanned from 9 to 12 hours per day. Despite ongoing psychotherapy with multiple providers with different orientations and approaches and numerous medication trials, he continued to experience significant anxiety, depression, ongoing self-harm, and problematic substance use of primarily cocaine and alcohol. Lee had been admitted, voluntarily, to several residential treatment programs for addiction, many of them featuring holistic health and wellness components with a length of stay of many months. Lee's family had considerable wealth from his father's inheritance and career as a venture capitalist. Lee's residential and outpatient psychotherapy and psychiatric care were paid for by his family who became increasingly concerned about his erratic behavior starting in early adolescence when his drug use began.

Lee was referred to an SDBT program at a private practice following a DUI charge. During the pretreatment screening process, he was asked to discontinue other forms of therapy while in DBT. He and his family begrudgingly agreed to discontinue Lee's other psychotherapy providers—he had ongoing meetings with a psychoanalyst and a therapeutic life coach—for the duration of Lee's time in DBT.

Lee also had chronic back and tailbone pain related to a diagnosis of scoliosis and relied on his family to manage and fund a range of rehabilitation and physical therapy regimens. At the time of intake, Lee relied on his mother for a range of self-management needs: coordinating with doctors and scheduling appointments, assisting Lee in following up with recommendations on managing chronic pain, and waking Lee up on a daily basis (often after 1 P.M. given that he was a "night owl" and would be up for most of the night gaming or on social media while intoxicated). His mother managed other activities of daily living, such as making sure he showered, brushed his teeth, and took his medications, all of which would drop off if his mother did not prompt him.

When Lee began SDBT, he was being supported by a cash allowance of $10,000 per month from his family. He would often exceed this amount with large purchases of clothing, devices, and gifts for friends, as well as funding his near daily cocaine use. Lee's finances were rarely called into question by his family, and no intervention was attempted with regard to his spending, other than his parents lamenting to him about his lack of structure and how undependable he was. They expressed concern about his cocaine use but did not seem to consider how unregulated access to money was a big factor in his obtaining the drug. In these conversations during pretreatment while the therapist was working to understand the environmental factors maintaining his dysfunctional behaviors, it was identified that Lee, the youngest of three siblings, would often be compared to his two older sisters who were highly accomplished in their academics and work in the field of finance and wealth management, just as their father had been. Lee was the "different" child and felt like an outsider on many levels. His parents would criticize his lack of motivation to pursue any "real-world" interests and express dissatisfaction and disappointment in him. The clinician found that engaging Lee in a discussion of his problems and goals during pretreatment sessions was a slow-moving process. Lee did speak clearly to problems in his family dynamics, however, including feeling like an outsider in his family on many levels and that he was "more emotional" than anyone in his family and that they "didn't get" him. Lee's clinician noted how his different emotional makeup stood out from that of his other family members while orienting to the biosocial theory of emotion dysregulation in these pretreatment sessions. The analogy of being "a rose in a tulip garden" was something Lee returned to and often referenced while discussing family dynamics in therapy.

Lee's SDBT year initially focused on commitment to closing the door to drug use: primarily cocaine, but also alcohol and prescription opiates. Stage 1 treatment also focused on learning skills to regulate and manage emotions in a way that would not involve drug use or self-harm. Lee was slow to engage in DBT after initial sporadic attendance; however, he began attending more regularly and meaningfully at month 3. At this point, he was experiencing a reduction in urges to use and self-harm. During this time, his mother began working with a DBT parent trainer at the recommendation of Lee's DBT therapist, so she was able to understand more of the biosocial theory of emotion dysregulation and was introduced to several skills to regulate her own behavior and emotions.

When DBT-ACES was first discussed at month 6 of SDBT, Lee thought about using drugs several times a week and would use an established skills plan to move through his cravings. While sobriety was largely maintained, he would also go back and forth between adding back the contact info for former drug dealers to his phone or following their accounts on social media, increasing the likelihood he would contact them for drugs.

When DBT-ACES was discussed, Lee noted that he had never had a job. His sisters began working in the finance field right after college by landing internships through their father's connections. One sister decided to quit in order to start a family. Lee was confused by his parents' wavering stance on his working. Often he was discouraged by his parents from applying for many jobs that they considered "menial" and "not worth it," yet they expressed disappointment in his lack of working and dim career prospects, particularly his lack of interest in finance. His family environment had set high expectations for lucrative work, yet there was not a lot of modeling or encouragement for him to take steps to get there.

Lee's DBT-ACES ambition was to develop a lucrative career and reduce financial dependency on his family. Self-sufficiency was also important in a range of other domains: He wanted to independently manage his chronic health condition and coordinate his own appointments, time, and day structure, and to observe limits with his mother, which triggered intense fear despite his tremendous love for her. Lee had lived in the same large metropolitan city his whole life and wanted to move to a different city to "get distance from the social influence" of his family. Additional components of his DBT-ACES ambition were to become more comfortable and self-accepting of being gay, to have a close group of gay friends in his community, and to find a loving and accepting life partner. He wanted to adopt several children and have a large family.

While starting the DBT-ACES pretreatment process at month 7 of SDBT, Lee was not at all clear what job he wanted to pursue as he had never considered an inspiring career path consistently. Lee would occasionally discuss pursuing a career as a school guidance counselor and spoke about having a glimmer of interest in this line of work since struggling in high school and receiving support from his guidance counselor. He found that when he brought this up with his parents, they would alternate between expressing support and then downplaying and minimizing the worth of his going back to school to get a degree in a field that was not lucrative. At times, his family also encouraged him to not work at all and to continue benefiting from their financial support, as other family members had also been encouraged to do.

When he started drafting the Career Plan in the DBT-ACES application, Lee would consider possible jobs, followed by rumination and worry about job prospects and whether employment was actually the path forward given his family resources. This rumination would be followed by intense urges to use. Discussing this with close friends yielded encouragement and validation, while discussion with family members would often leave him feeling more emotionally dysregulated.

Fear and social expectations were functioning to reinforce avoidance of employment and goals of self-sufficiency. Yet at the same time, Lee felt that his relationship with his family was becoming more and more fractured, even with his mother's DBT parent coaching, and he desperately wanted to get distance and space from them. However, his financial dependence made that difficult. He also began to gain awareness of the biosocial theory and the transaction between invalidating environment and emotional vulnerability, and found that making changes to his family's pattern of invalidation would require, at the very least, observing limits by him having his own funds. He decided to apply to DBT-ACES and continue to observe his goals and the emotions that they prompted, mainly fear, shame, and sadness.

During this time in SDBT, Lee continued working with his therapist on understanding invalidating influences and the impact on his behavior, as well as observing limits with his family and managing the contingencies that were present in the day-to-day events of their home life. His mother joined for part of several individual sessions, and in one session Lee used his interpersonal skills (DEAR MAN) to request that she no longer wake him up, coordinate his appointments, and follow up on the range of self-management activities that she currently oversaw.

As part of working to observe limits with his family and focusing on relevant QOL issues, Lee's therapist also provided ongoing validation as Lee worked toward accepting and affirming his identity as a gay man. Validation was used to acknowledge and support Lee's process of understanding and grieving his sense of otherness and separateness from his immediate family, stemming from his different emotional makeup (he would feel negative emotions more strongly and take longer to recover) and wildly different interests. Lee experienced his family as driven and accomplished, whereas he was not. He experienced both of his sisters as very supportive of him being gay since he had come out to the family 2 years earlier at age 21. In contrast, his parents had both shown lukewarm support of his sexual orientation, and he would often experience intense fear, shame, and sadness when it was a topic of discussion between them, even in passing. In SDBT, he began growing acceptance that this was one more way in which he was an outsider from his tight-knit family unit—his primary social influence—and began allowing the grief and disappointment that were part of the process of acceptance.

As the SDBT year progressed, the therapist continued to target increased participation in social activities and volunteering through the use of the Normative Productivity contingency and building in structured, scheduled, and social weekly Getting Active hours. As of month 8, Lee began volunteering at a drop-in center for at-risk LGBTQ+ youth in his city. He would often stay for several hours after his shift with other volunteers and staff members. This was a relatively structured, scheduled, and social volunteer activity, and it served to boost Lee's mood and sense of confidence and purpose. He noticed less cravings to use drugs several weeks into the volunteer work, and urges to self-harm had been largely absent for months. He was also able to expand his social circle to include many friends who had shared values, something for which he had longed for many years.

Lee's therapist felt that this behavioral shaping represented great progress. Volunteer work was selected and implemented independently from his family, which was a huge step forward on his self-management recovery goals. His mother was managing self-care activities, appointments, and waking him up less and less. Lee and his therapist would appreciate the progress and celebrate the success while acknowledging that, in order to build a life that was more meaningful, he would need to approach settings where he had more accountability. The focus of SDBT at this time was largely on problem solving and shaping: creating a calendar on his device, organizing to-do tasks, and independently building a more consistent sleep–wake cycle. Approaching self-management goals often prompted shame and sadness and "comparison thoughts" to others. When he experienced shame, Lee's typical response would be increased self-invalidation, negative self-talk, and having urges to quit commitments and withdraw socially. He would hide from most social situations and continue to avoid, albeit with a sadness and lethargy that drugs had often helped to suppress. He experienced these times as more misery than ever before.

Lee and his therapist worked together to gradually expose him to shame-provoking situations while increasing mindfulness of current emotion that allowed him to ride waves of shame. In-session and out-of-session, Lee's tendency to look away and become quiet and withdrawn were blocked, and he was encouraged to stay mindful, share nonjudgmentally about his reaction to the tasks ahead, and reflect his therapist's response of support, acceptance, and lack of ostracization. The therapist would provide extensive validation in the context of him riding the wave of shame or acting opposite by sharing what qualities of himself or his behaviors prompted shame, and Lee was coached to observe and describe the therapist's responses as a way to counter the shame response and block the shame spiral. The therapeutic relationship and Lee's interactions with certain friends were also opportunities to practice exposure and opposite action to shame.

Lee submitted his DBT-ACES application in his 10th month of SDBT and started DBT-ACES immediately after graduating from SDBT. He wanted to "keep the momentum going" and was concerned that a break in therapy would leave him vulnerable to sliding backward toward substance use.

At month 4 of DBT-ACES—right up against the deadline to start Work as Therapy or take a therapy vacation—Lee applied to and got a job working at a clothing boutique, a position that he heard about from a friend who knew the owner. Soon after starting work, his manager provided the feedback that he was good with customers and coworkers interpersonally, but was on track to be written up due to ongoing lateness. The negative feedback about his lateness prompted intense guilt and shame, which Lee worked to problem-solve in individual therapy sessions. After initial strategies to reduce shame, noted above, he recovered from this feedback with a more determined and mindful approach to managing his time so that he would consistently be on time to work. After several weeks of being on time, the therapist worked to help Lee take in the evidence to support the notion that he was a productive and respected coworker, based on the positive feedback he received from his manager and getting more seniority with work scheduling, which had been a major goal.

Individual sessions focused on Lee applying skills to excel at his current job while also searching for a job that better fit his personality and values. Though Lee was now employed, he felt neutral about his job and did not look forward to his shifts as he had with his volunteer work at the LGBTQ+ youth drop-in center. Not only was he around other like-minded people with similar values within the same LGBTQ+ community, but assessment revealed that the fast-paced and highly stimulating environment of a drop-in center setting was where he felt most comfortable.

The skill of Community Mapping from the Establishing and Re-Evaluating Relationships DBT Next Steps skills module was an integral part of Lee choosing to expand his social network to include individuals with shared interests and approach new settings where he wouldn't encounter drug use. Other skills from this module helped Lee to build more social connections that were key goals for him. His focus on the Diving Into New Relationships skill provided a framework for preparing to find satisfying relationships, as well as strategies for how to find them and behaviors to increase their quality and the connection. The Re-Establishing Existing Relationships skill helped Lee to decide what past fragile, avoided, lost, or damaged relationships to resurrect. This involved Lee observing his limits to get more clarity on the friendships that "fell through the cracks" and the behaviors of his friends that were worth tolerating, using the "ideal community map" to guide the process. Lee consulted his Wise Mind and drew the conclusion that there was minimal room in his life for the people with whom he had used drugs or who had relied on Lee to buy their drugs, as well as people who failed to provide support or allyship to Lee as an out gay man. Lee was able to build more satisfying and supportive social connections, and also observe his limits and develop more mindful distance from several family members.

His Career Goal in his DBT-ACES application had focused on getting his degree and working toward a career as a guidance counselor. This had been informed by his experience working with a guidance counselor in high school, volunteering at the youth drop-in center, and being drawn to informal mentorship opportunities. With this course in mind, individual sessions focused on cueing him to increase opposite action and mindfulness as activation, and continuing to throw himself into his job at the clothing boutique until he was able to problem-solve and land a job more closely aligned with his goal of becoming a guidance counselor, where his Career Development hours would ultimately be focused. Six months into DBT-ACES, he was hired as an administrative assistant in a college advising center.

At the time of Lee's DBT-ACES graduation, he had accumulated enough savings in his recently opened checking account so that he could move out and live independently. Although he ultimately decided to remain living with his family for the time being and continue to live off his monthly allowance, he felt a sense of competence and confidence about having the option to move out and live independently. His family relationships had changed quite a bit after Lee's emphasis on self-management recovery goals and managing all aspects of self-care, scheduling, and managing medical appointments. This was due, in part, to Lee working with his therapist to implement a contingency management plan whereby he would reinforce his mother when she would hold back from trying to coordinate his self-management activities. He had started dating and attending meet-ups for sober gay men in his community. While this had not led to a sense of community and connection yet, Lee had a balanced perspective that it was an important step to expand opportunities for social connection in places and settings where he had commonalities and shared values with others in the room. He was able to continue to go on dates and attend these social meetings by cheerleading himself on with the belief that the more he put himself out there, the more likely friendships or relationships were bound to happen. He had embraced an approach of opposite action to shame and fear that moved him forward in many domains in his life: leisure, personal growth, health management, relationships and community building, as well as work.

As these two case examples illustrate, DBT Next Steps includes targeted skills training, reinforcement of adaptive behavior, cognitive modification, and unique contingency management and exposure-based strategies that function to initiate and maintain employment and self-sufficiency behaviors—as well as to proactively structure one's environment to facilitate employment and self-sufficiency. We will now move on to Part II of the book, where we will discuss adaptations to SDBT strategies that are critical to mobilizing the client to block avoidance and decide what Next Steps they have to take, learn new skills, and use exposure and contingency management to drag new behavior to achieve their life worth living goals.

PART II

DBT NEXT STEPS STRATEGIES

CHAPTER 4

Recovery Goals

Bringing Clarity and Precision to Quality-of-Life Targets

We begin Part II with DBT targets specific to Next Steps. As previously discussed, DBT Next Steps uses the same general hierarchy as SDBT: (1) life-threatening behaviors, (2) TIB, (3) QOL-interfering behaviors, and (4) increasing DBT skills use and competence. DBT Next Steps comes into the picture when the behavioral dyscontrol targets have been addressed and the focus has moved to the actions that need to be taken to build a life worth living and address the skills deficits, contingencies, and avoidance of feared cues that hold back the client.

One issue we observe over and over is that targeting is harder the lower down the hierarchy you get. At the top of the hierarchy—when someone has cut themself or had a spike of suicidal ideation, missed a group, or used meth—there is a clear problem behavior, often indicative of dyscontrol. When there is a specific incident, it is easier to chain and to work on replacing it with other more adaptive behaviors. As the therapist and client resolve these high targets and move down into QOL-interfering targets that aren't specific instances of dyscontrol, it can become murkier. For example, a client's goal is to return to college and find a new group of friends, yet they are currently living at home with their parents and don't have a job or independent income. What is the QOL-interfering behavior you are targeting? Sometimes this is a question of getting adequately specific, such as determining if there is a behavior to increase or decrease or a stimulus control problem where the behavior is reasonable but not in the situations where it occurs (e.g., screaming at the TV during a football game vs. screaming at your roommates). Even then, however, clients are often missing key skills, are getting reinforced for dysfunctional behavior, inadequately reinforced for functional behavior, or are avoiding. Thus, the problems continue. So, the dyad jumps to another behaviorally defined target to try instead, and that doesn't work. As this process repeats itself, both the client and therapist can grow discouraged.

To address this, Marsha Linehan asked the Harborview team a very good question: What are the typical QOL behaviors that interfere with financial independence, strong social networks, self-sufficiency, and other life worth living goals? We developed a list and then decided to reverse them from QOL-interfering behaviors to their opposite: goals to be achieved. We call these Recovery Goals because they are key targets to achieve what most clients would call recovery from psychiatric disability and are core to achieving their life worth living goals. Recovery Goals include goals that are specific to living wage employment like choosing a career path, to self-sufficiency like budgeting time and money, to social and leisure activities like having friends whose values align with yours, as well as key interpersonal and emotion regulation goals that are critical for long-term success, such as tolerating difficult coworkers and remaining regulated even when provoked. This isn't a complete list—most therapists and clients will likely identify others—but it is a comprehensive starting point that helps therapists and clients decide where to focus in building a new life. The remainder of this chapter will review and explain each of the Recovery Goals.

Description of Recovery Goals

Meaningful Work

The first set of Recovery Goals relates to finding, starting, and following a career path that matters to the client. As described in Part I of this book, we have found that a job or career path is very important to the majority of clients for many different reasons. For some clients, the only point of a career is the money, so they can do the things they aspire to or enjoy. Some have a deep love for or commitment to something around which they want to build their career, such as helping people, a scientific or engineering breakthrough, or the arts. Some clients want to travel and see new places, so their goal is a career that pays the bills and still leaves enough time and money to see the world. Other clients want freedom and independence from family or the social welfare system, so a career is about making enough money to be financially independent or have a home of their own. Most clients see job or career as status within their family or culture when their goal is to fulfill expectations; as an answer to the question "What do you do?" or relief from pressure or disappointment from their family.

Two often undervalued aspects of work (and school) are socialization and structure. As is often quoted, having friends at work makes job satisfaction higher. The opposite is also true: Jobs and education are pathways to interaction with a large number of people. People are in contact with each other over time, which builds trust and connection. This leads to a range of relationships, from the most casual acquaintances who share a copy machine or a workspace to "best friends forever." When a client's (or therapist's) social needs are met at work, they can often enjoy their alone time at home much more deeply—appreciate it for the solitude, quiet, or rest that it can be—and this results in less loneliness, including for people who are single or living alone.

Another core benefit of work and school is structure and contingencies that reinforce adaptive behavior. Life on disability can be very hard—a whole day, a whole week, stretches out before you, and it can take a lot of effort to fill the time with meaningful and enjoyable activities if you have to plan what you are doing each day, all day, every day. If you are feeling emotional or physical pain, you have to make an effort to find something to be mindful of over and over again, rather than having work or school activities that take your mind off the pain.

Without structure and the consequences for not following it, procrastination can be a constant companion. You could grocery shop now, but also in an hour, or this afternoon, or this evening. Ironically, this makes the effort greater than when you are busy with work or school and your time to go to the store is limited to 3–4 free hours during the week. For something about which you have ambivalence, you can find yourself in a vicious cycle of fear, shame, and procrastination. When procrastination is the "same as emotion" behavior for fear and shame, the more you feel fear and shame, the more you procrastinate, which further triggers fear and shame. Thus, procrastination deepens the ambivalence, fear, and shame and digs an ever-deeper hole of avoidance and isolation.

It is for all of these reasons that work and school should always be considered for life worth living goals and for QOL on the target hierarchy. There are always exceptions, chief among them responsibilities in the home and family that function in the same way. Parents or grandparents who care for children and the home are often provided with as much or more status, social life, and structure as those working or in school—if not as much money and independence. Adults caring for elderly or disabled family members or volunteering in a time-consuming but important way in their community can also achieve these same benefits. If the question, therefore, is "why not" work or school, then it helps to consider if there are alternatives that serve these same core functions.

The specific Recovery Goals related to Meaningful Work are:

- Choose a career path to employment knowing its fit with your Wise Mind values and talents as well as the practical issues of pay, health insurance, leave and retirement benefits, hours, shift times, required training or certification, and routes to advancement.
- Demonstrate capability to financially support yourself (and your family) in your chosen career without psychiatric disability payments or partner's/family's income.
- Demonstrate capability to financially support yourself (and your family) in at least one fallback job without psychiatric disability payments or partner's/family's income (if needed).
- Have sufficient health insurance to maintain health care and medications.
- Exhibit better than 90% follow-through at work on attendance, being on time, appropriate dress and manner, following directions, and job tasks.

Interpersonal Proficiency

As we discuss with our clients regularly, most people's success at work (and life) is based on their Interpersonal Proficiency. The ability to do the job is surprisingly less important. For clients who have been emotionally dysregulated and interpersonally sensitive for most of their lives, it can be hard to understand what is needed to become someone with whom people want to work and hang out. The following Recovery Goals are key for establishing Interpersonal Proficiency:

- Become interpersonally easy to work/be with—even with difficult people and during stressful times.
- Demonstrate the capability to regulate emotional expression and actions and find Wise Mind in all interpersonal situations—even with difficult people and during stressful times.

- Know your Wise Mind personal limits and act on them with yourself, employer, friends, family, colleagues, and members of your community.
- Receive praise, raises, promotions, and offers for more desirable jobs and roles within your community.

Life Outside Work

With Meaningful Work and Interpersonal Proficiency, some parts of Life Outside Work will naturally sort themselves out. Of course, some people will become workaholics to avoid the challenges of life outside of work, or because work and school is such fun. People also differ in terms of their sociability. Extroverts benefit from multiple friends and social engagements, and introverts may be deeply content with being part of something meaningful to them and one or two close friends. Keeping these things in mind, we have developed Life Outside Work Recovery Goals to capture this dialectic while holding to the importance of supportive and meaningful human connection (often the same person or place can serve multiple goals):

- Have at least a couple of local and/or long-distance friends whose values align with yours.
- Have at least one person or group for casual interactions (e.g., lunchroom, church, coffee, movie, sports event, volunteer organization).
- Have at least one close support with whom you experience intimacy and discuss private issues who is not your therapist.
- Have at least one local person or group that would notice you were not around and would take action to find you.
- Be an active member of an organized recreational activity that is either fun or meaningful and not related to mental health (e.g., volunteer organization, church, sports teams, hiking, fishing, Spanish lessons, ballroom dancing).
- Disengage from relationships with family members that are ineffective or destructive.
- Disengage or end friendships that are ineffective or destructive.
- Choose relationships based on evidence that they are compatible with your lifestyle, needs, and values.
- Take steps to find an effective and rewarding romantic relationship (if desired).

Emotional Proficiency

By achieving behavioral control, many but not all DBT clients have also achieved Emotional Proficiency. The level of proficiency demanded by work and school—not to mention relationships with "high-quality" friends and romantic partners, children, and aging parents—exceeds what it takes just to be able to hold it together. With that in mind, we have developed three Emotional Proficiency Recovery Goals:

- Be able to experience negative emotions building, staying, and falling mindfully—not avoiding, rushing them along, or mentally moving into a different moment.
- Be able to experience positive emotions building, staying, and falling mindfully—not avoiding, rushing them along, or mentally moving into a different moment.
- Be able to reduce problematic emotions effectively and fast enough to prevent them from leading to problems.

Self-Management

Last, but not least, is Self-Management: targets that are critical for self-sufficiency in the present, but also to sustain a new life into the future. Most clients will have a handle on one or more of these even before coming to DBT, but there will usually be a few that they are less comfortable with. These should be the focus of treatment to reach the Next Steps. The Self-Management Recovery Goals are:

- Have an effective method for managing your monthly budget and one-time expenses (e.g., new tires) so you stay within your income.
- Have sufficient emergency fund savings to cover 3 months of living expenses in case you lose your job.
- Have an effective method of saving for things you would enjoy.
- Have an effective method for getting out of debt or reducing debt to a reasonable level.
- Have an effective method for managing your time in line with your Wise Mind values.
- Have an effective method for managing your time that gets key things done on time.
- Have an effective method for managing your time that balances work, leisure, household, and downtime.
- Have an effective method of preventing illness and psychiatric symptoms from impacting your functioning.
- Have an effective method of managing chronic illness or pain to minimize its impact on your QOL.

Targeting with Recovery Goals

As in SDBT, therapists adhere to the treatment hierarchy, which means that suicidal or therapy-interfering behavior is given priority when it appears; however in DBT Next Steps, the majority of treatment is focused on these Recovery Goals. Recovery Goals are targeted in the order agreed upon by the client and individual therapist. We recommend that clients quarterly reassess their progress on these targets using the Self-Assessment of Recovery Goals form (found in the companion volume for clients, *DBT Next Steps Skills Handouts*), and that this is reviewed by the therapist and the consultation team to assure the individual therapist is targeting effectively.

In a comprehensive DBT-ACES program, other QOL-interfering behaviors are treated only when Recovery Goal targets have been sufficiently addressed. However, if integrating DBT Next Steps into existing DBT therapy, when to target these Recovery Goals versus other issues (e.g., traumatic experiencing or chronic pain) is more complicated, depending on how fully the therapy has focused on building a life worth living through overcoming avoidance and pursuing positive opportunities. If this is the focus, it is important to consider whether jumping on and off of the Recovery Goals—either by the client, the therapist, or both—is functioning as avoidance, or whether there is differential reinforcement for the Recovery Goals as opposed to other issues. As with all things in DBT, our goal is to support the client's ultimate goals, and the therapist should be mindful of and vigilant about targeting. Otherwise, DBT Next Steps will wander around without a clear outcome to show for it.

For example, clients with social anxiety frequently engage in avoidance behaviors that interfere with both obtaining employment and making friends. Socially anxious behaviors then become a focus of DBT Next Steps individual therapy to achieve the employment and social network goals. However, if social anxiety was not related to a DBT Next Steps Recovery Goal, it might be best postponed until the Recovery Goals are substantially met. As another example, substance abuse is a frequent QOL-interfering behavior. In SDBT, an assessment is made whether the client's substance abuse is a life-threatening behavior and/or TIB, or a key factor controlling whether a top target occurs. Substance abuse is only addressed if it is a key controlling factor until the life-threatening behavior and TIBs are in substantial control. At that point, substance abuse may become a QOL treatment target of its own. Similar principles exist as you move to DBT Next Steps, although at that point, clients have stopped most crisis- and therapy-interfering behaviors (and the use of substances to the extent that it causes these behaviors). The DBT therapist prioritizes targeting remaining substance use problems if they relate to the Recovery Goals. For instance, drinking too much the night before work, causing one to be late or unable to attend; drinking to reduce social anxiety when it is not acceptable to the friends with whom the client is hanging out; and use or possession of illegal substances that interfere with obtaining a job or with school performance can all be addressed as part of the Recovery Goals. Discussion with the DBT consultation team is often key in deciding these targeting dilemmas.

Using the Diary Card to Track Recovery Goals for Individual Psychotherapy

Given the potentially large number of Recovery Goals to target, the DBT therapist and client need to decide which to focus on. Some can be ignored because the client has already achieved them. Some are related to the Career Activities and Work as Therapy contingencies and will have to be targeted early in treatment to get meaningful work off the ground. Thus, some will need to be put off.

The Standard DBT Diary Card includes tracking Normative Productive Hours (see Appendix 1 of the *DBT Next Steps Skills Handouts* volume for a template) given the benefit of increasing structured, scheduled social activities in Standard DBT. The DBT Next Steps Diary Card is another mechanism to help keep the individual therapist and client moving in the direction of behavioral activation and Recovery Goals (see Figure 4.1 and Appendix 2 of *DBT Next Steps Skills Handouts* for an example). The Diary Card is divided into two sections, as is typical of SDBT: The targets to track and steps toward Recovery Goals are listed on the front, with DBT skills to practice on the back. The difference in the DBT Next Steps Diary Card is that, on the top, suicidal urges and behaviors are moved to the bottom of the list with open boxes to write in individual targets. This deemphasizes suicidal behavior without removing it from self-monitoring.

The target boxes are empty, as these should be developed by the individual therapist and client together. To develop Diary Card ratings, follow these steps:

1. Agree with the client on at least one behavior to increase or decrease that reflects the Recovery Goal of interest.
2. Define it behaviorally (topography, intensity, frequency, duration) sufficiently that you can make a daily rating that is either yes/no, number of times, 0–5 rating, and so forth. This goes in the Actions section.

DBT Next Steps Diary Card

Name: ______________________ **Date:** ________ **Number days completed:** ______

	Day of the Week							
URGES								
	Suicidal ideation							
	Self-harm							
ACTIONS								
	Self-harm							
EMOTIONS	Love							
	Joy							
	Anger							
	Sadness							
	Fear							
	Shame							

Primary ambition(s) (including but maybe greater than ambition presented in skills-training group):

Agenda Items and Notes for Session

DBT Next Steps Skills and Strategies to Achieve Your Ambition(s) and Recovery Goals:								
Home-work	Worked on Check-In Action Step.							
	Interacted with DBT Next Steps material.							
	Worked on assignments for this week.							
Living Wage Employment and Interpersonal Proficiency	On time and stayed full-session at work/school.							
	Percentage of day followed schedule/time map.							
	Did you stay regulated at work/school today?							
	Did you use reducing vulnerability skills today?							
	Did you use Wise Mind to balance your priorities with others' demands?							
	Did you presume nonjudgmental explanation of others' behavior at work/school today?							
	Did you avoid something important today?							
	No. of times GIVE with new/important person?							
	Describe if/how GIVE was experienced by those with whom you work or attend school:							
Building Community	Did you meaningfully reach out today?							
	Describe if/how GIVE was experienced by friends, family, or partner:							
	Did you spend time with people you like and care about? What did you do?							
	Did you effectively attend a social event with GIVE? What did you do?							
Self-sufficient	Bills paid up:							
	Money paid toward debt:							
	Money new debt incurred:							
	Money put toward savings:							

From your calendar, please note the following for past week:

Hours worked W2 job: ______

Hours of other paid job: ______

Hours of unpaid job in field: ______

Hours attended school: ______

Hours other scheduled activities: ______

Total hours: ______

No. of applications submitted: ______

No. of interviews: ______

No. of contacts asked about jobs: ______

Total: ______

(continued)

FIGURE 4.1. DBT Next Steps Diary Card.

DBT Next Steps Diary Card *(page 2 of 2)*

Emotionally Proficient	DBT skill of the week:							
	Experienced fully a wave of emotion:							
	Regulated quickly enough to be fully effective:							

Describe efforts toward deadlines with specifics (e.g., dates, who):

Standard DBT Skills—Check the boxes below for each day you worked on each skill.								
	DAY OF THE WEEK							
	DATE							
Mindfulness	**Wise Mind**							
	Observe (just notice)							
	Describe (put words on)							
	Participate (enter into the experience)							
	Nonjudgmental (not good nor bad)							
	One-mindfully (only the present moment)							
	Effectiveness (focus on what works)							
Interpersonal Effectiveness	**Figure out interpersonal priorities**							
	DEAR (Describe, Express, Assert, Reinforce)							
	MAN—Mindful (Broken Record, Ignore Attacks), Appear Confident, Negotiate							
	GIVE (Gentle, Interested, Validate, Easy Manner)							
	FAST (Fair, No Apologies, Stick to Values, Truthful)							
	Self-Validation							
	Finding/Getting People to Like You							
Emotion Regulation	**Observing and Describing Emotions**							
	Opposite Action							
	Check the Facts							
	Problem Solving							
	Accumulate Positives short term							
	Accumulate Positives long term							
	Build Mastery							
	Cope Ahead (plan + mental rehearsal)							
	PLEASE							
	Mindfulness of Current Emotion (a.k.a. Ride the Wave)							
Distress Tolerance	**STOP**							
	TIPP—Temperature (dive), Intense Exercise, Paced Breathing, PMR							
	Pros and Cons							
	Distract (ACCEPTS)							
	Self-Soothe (five senses)							
	IMPROVE							
	Dialectical Abstinence							
	Radical Acceptance/Turn the Mind							
	Willingness/Half-Smile/Willing Hands							
	Mindfulness of Current Thoughts							

NUMBER DAYS COMPLETED DIARY CARD: ______

FIGURE 4.1. *(continued)*

3. It can also be helpful to have an observation/urge rating to do that Action (or avoid that Action) each day on the standard 0–5 scale.
4. Often, a rating of life worth living experience (e.g., feeling confident, feeling loved, feeling connected) that changing a behavior would achieve is useful in the Observation/Urges section.

For example, if the client and therapist are targeting the Recovery Goal of having a local group that would miss you if you didn't show up, the Diary Card ratings might include:

- An Action rating each day of Went to Volunteer Group (yes/no)
- A rating of urge to volunteer (0–5) or, by contrast, social anxiety (0–5)
- A rating of your goal for volunteering might be a Sense of Belonging (0–5) or Someone Called/Texted Me (yes/no)

At the bottom of the DBT Next Steps Diary Card are ratings that attempt to behaviorally capture the Recovery Goals. There are a lot of ratings here, so it is important to decide if a specific client should delete, "grey out," or cross out ratings that are not immediately relevant or already achieved. Many clients can or want to rate the whole list, though, so also be sure not to fragilize. Rewording a rating to be clearer for you or the client is appropriate—the goal is to capture the meaning of the Recovery Goals in a useful fashion. As in any DBT context, the client should see themself and their therapy reflected in the Diary Card. Extraneous ratings that aren't meaningful don't add anything and might detract a lot.

Recovery Goals Self-Assessment

The Self-Assessment of Recovery Goals form is used periodically (generally every 3 months) to help the client and individual therapist manage the large number of Recovery Goals and stay on track. The self-assessment lists each of the Recovery Goals, and the client is asked to rate each on a 7-point scale of competence. The scale is modeled on the SDBT skills rating from the SDBT Diary Card and captures how well that Recovery Goal has been achieved and integrated into the client's behavioral repertoire. Following this, the client is asked to list what they are responsible for as this addresses both their normative and productive activity and social connections from a personalized angle.

It is helpful to start with the Self-Assessment of Recovery Goals as a pretreatment approach for DBT Next Steps when the client has gained behavioral control and is ready to move on to building up their life. In a comprehensive DBT-ACES program, this is embedded in a formal application, but the self-assessment can be used as a tool on its own to help a client think through what is involved in DBT Next Steps and how it relates to them. To facilitate this, clients are asked to make their initial Recovery Goal self-assessment ratings both for the time they entered DBT and for the present.

If a client is completing the DBT Next Steps skills-training group, the Self-Assessment of Recovery Goals appears twice in the skills assignments as the final assignment of two of the modules. These self-assessments ask only about the present and include a second rating of whether or not that Recovery Goal is a focus of the client's current individual therapy. These self-assessments are reviewed during skills-training group and turned in to the group leaders who pass them along to the individual therapists for review. This gives the individual therapists an opportunity to see if they agree with the client's ratings of progress and whether or not they agree on what they are targeting in session.

As noted in Chapter 2, the DBT consultation team should block about 30 minutes of a team meeting to review the self-assessments and help the individual therapists be sure they are maximizing the effectiveness of their targeting and troubleshoot as needed. The DBT consultation team should work hard at the dialectical balance of letting the primary therapist be a primary therapist and make the final decision while also challenging therapists when their targeting seems to avoid difficult targets, when they are leaving out important targets, when they are assuming something has been achieved that has not been, and the like. "Therapy for the therapist" principles should be followed, remembering that this client is the same client all the team members are treating by treating the individual therapist in a consultation team.

CHAPTER 5

Skills Training

Learning New Skills and Lots of Practice

Skills-Training Goals

The primary goal of the DBT Next Steps Skills Curriculum is for clients to learn to be their own therapist, at least as it relates to general mental health stability. Specific capabilities include being able to:

- Mix and match skills; that is, to assess a problem and match skills to it, not just see a skill and match problems to it (as in SDBT skills training).
- Understand explicitly what they experience implicitly in individual therapy, including behavioral assessment, reinforcement, goal setting, problem solving, troubleshooting, cognitive restructuring, and dialectics, and be able to apply them with themselves and their environment.
- Understand explicitly the steps needed to create their own social support system and effectively interact with people at work, new and established friends, and treatment providers.
- Develop proficiency in these skills through repeated practice.

We think of this as analogous to the difference between undergraduate and graduate training: In undergraduate school, you learn subject matter in theory, and in graduate school, you learn to apply what you have learned in structured practice, to become a practitioner yourself, and to teach others (e.g., the Career Activities, Work as Therapy, and Check-In for DBT Next Steps are like practica and internships in graduate school).

To improve capacity to achieve Next Steps, a new DBT Next Steps skills-training curriculum linked to the Recovery Goals has been created. The DBT Next Steps curriculum includes:

- More applied versions of the SDBT skills
- Other CBT skills such as goal setting, problem solving, and contingency management
- Specific interpersonal skills to function effectively at work and with health care providers, and to establish oneself in a supportive community outside of one focused on mental health
- Strategies to overcome the typical problems of psychiatrically disabled individuals, including rigid or perfectionistic thinking, time mismanagement, anxiety, anger, and depression
- Balance of acceptance-based skills modules (e.g., Applications of Mindfulness) with change-based skills modules (e.g., Managing Emotions Effectively)

Detailed lesson plans for the DBT Next Steps skills can be found in Part IV of this clinician's guide, and the handouts and assignments for clients can be found in our companion book, *DBT Next Steps Skills Handouts.*

DBT Next Steps Skills-Training Modules

DBT Next Steps skills modules are designed to take 1 month each, beginning with the first week of the month. The curriculum is based on 4 weeks, but in months with 5 weeks, the group leaders can decide what material is worth expanding on or teach related material from another source. In that case, group leaders can make up new assignments, repeat an assignment, or give an assignment vacation.

There are six skills modules, which can be offered once or twice. We have generally offered each module twice so that, as in SDBT, clients go through the skills curriculum twice in 1 year. This may be more than is needed for younger clients who are used to school environments and learning skills. For instance, an adolescent or young adult client could complete their standard DBT program in 16 weeks or 6 months, and then finish the DBT Next Steps curriculum in 6 months. This might be particularly relevant for a young person who fell off track due to depression or increased self-harm or addiction, leading them to be out of sync with their peers on Next Steps like college or first jobs. A faster, 6-month trip through DBT Next Steps, after they have learned to control these behaviors, is a great opportunity for them to catch up.

While the order of modules is not fixed, this order has been effective in our program and is the order in which the modules are presented in Part IV of this book:

- Perfectionism versus Reinforcement
- Establishing and Re-Evaluating Relationships
- Time Management
- Managing Emotions Effectively
- Succeeding after DBT
- Applications of Mindfulness

There are client handouts and teaching points for each module. In Part IV, the teaching points for each module are described week by week and linked to the handouts in *DBT Next Steps Skills Handouts.*

Client handouts for each module start with a syllabus sheet that lists the topics for each week and the assignment associated with each teaching topic. Participants are, therefore, pre-informed of the assignments and are expected to independently keep up with the material even if they miss a week (just like they would be expected to do in college or at work). In fact, we recommend that clients pursuing DBT Next Steps behave as if attending a college course or at a training at work with their supervisor present when they attend skills training. They should dress appropriately for their career plans (which might differ significantly depending on career path and culture). The group leaders can coach clients with regard to this expectation, set contingencies, and reinforce effective behavior.

DBT Next Steps Assignments

For DBT Next Step skills, the word "assignments" is used in lieu of "homework" or "worksheets" because this word is more general to work, not just school contexts. Assignments in DBT Next Steps should always be completed in writing ahead of time, as this is the expectation of most job and school programs and leads to a more thorough understanding of the material. Also, writing notes during class and review of their assignments provide the client with a completed notebook and relevant correct examples to go back and review in the future.

Assignments are expected to be completed for each week, even if the client missed the class or the assignment was done but not written down for a previous class. Our goal is to introduce a range of skills that may be helpful now and to which the client can return in the months and years after graduation when a problem in that area arises. Complete, written assignments that are corrected as needed during assignment review ensure that the clients (1) practice each skill that we teach so they are sure they understand them and are able to ask questions and get corrections, (2) know what the pros and cons of that skill are, and (3) have correct notes in their skills book for reference after graduation.

Clients are oriented to the need for complete, written assignments as they are oriented to DBT Next Steps and the skills-training class. Clients are also oriented to treat these assignments as they would at work or in college—do assignments completely, on time, neatly, and be ready to discuss. If they do not complete assignments on time, clients are informed that, as in a work or college situation, they need to take the initiative to catch the skills co-leader at an appropriate time (e.g., during a break, before class) to show them their now completed assignments and to ask any questions (this role is for the skills co-leader, not the skills leader in charge of primary teaching). If the client did the assignment and did not write it down, they can report their practice during group but will still be asked to write it out for review by the skills co-leader at the next group.

The skills co-leader is not expected to have to chase down clients to obtain their assignments. At the same time, the skills co-leader should maintain at least a general track record of how many assignments the clients are behind.

If the client is four or more assignments behind, they are suspended from the DBT Next Steps skills class until they are caught up. Generally, if clients come to group but are too many assignments behind to attend, we recommend that such clients be asked to sit in the lobby and complete assignments until they are caught up and then join group as soon as they are less than four assignments behind. Unlike the four-miss or 24-hour arbitrary rules where the withdrawal of therapy is for a fixed period (the length of the therapy contract according to the four-miss rule and 24 hours in the case of the 24-hour rule), the duration of suspension for being behind on assignments is under the control of the individual. This introduces a reinforcement aspect, as with the "therapy vacation" in SDBT. Clients are welcomed back to therapy as soon as they are less than four assignments behind, and the co-leader will offer coaching to get completely caught up. Leaders and group members will all be glad to see the client back and will share that verbally and nonverbally, which supplies additional positive reinforcement for getting the work done. This TIB should also be targeted by the individual therapist.

This is a dialectic for co-leaders who aren't naturally inclined to tracking details: They must both be on top of whether folks are behind and not get burned out by tracking such clients. One synthesis we recommend is sending a group email or information sheet to the individual therapists listing the clients who did not complete their assignment (a sample template of the group email is included in this book's Appendix A and a blank template is included in Appendix B). Another synthesis is to put as much pressure as possible on the clients to track their late assignments themselves, like prompting them to say how many they are behind as they head into break. The goal is to find a synthesis for your team that meets DBT principles and makes assignment tracking as painless as possible.

If clients have questions about getting themselves to do the assignment or have complaints about the assignment, they should take these to the individual therapist who functions as a private coach—just as we would not want the client to bring complaints or statements of general inability to their boss or professor during a meeting or class. They should primarily practice their interpersonal skills (GIVE, DEAR MAN, and FAST skills) with their skills leaders as they would use them with their boss or teacher at college—skillfully.

In class, the review of assignments should be for correctness, completeness, and mindfulness. When the skills co-leader reviews past assignments at break or another opportunity, the guideline is the same; time may not allow for a detailed review, so the priority is completeness and general correctness. As in SDBT, in-class review of assignments is a continuation of the teaching, not just to confirm assignments are complete. It is an opportunity for additional teaching to fine-tune clients' understanding and increase their troubleshooting with the skill. The goal of DBT Next Steps skills training is that the client has sufficient competency with each skill taught to be able to use it independently and effectively on their own, to be able to troubleshoot when their use of the skill is problematic, and to remember it or have a reference point to refer to after graduation.

It is important for skills group leaders to reinforce effective assignments and, in particular, ambitious or thorough assignments and creativity. Generally, this is done with validation, praise, irreverence, or another light strategy that is an effective reinforcer for that client. One goal of DBT Next Steps is to learn how to "read a room" and be able to see what reinforces others and use reinforcers flexibly with different people. Now is a good chance for skills leaders to model this skill.

Several assignments throughout the year involve the clients interviewing or role-playing situations with their individual therapist. Be sure that the individual therapists are oriented and committed to doing such assignments before assigning them. It is also helpful if the skills leaders remind individual therapists when such assignments are upcoming so individual therapists can pace sessions accordingly.

It is helpful if skills leaders have a system of communicating with individual therapists about attendance, assignment completion, and the behavioral effectiveness of their clients so the individual therapists can help clients be successful in group. We use our secure email system or a worksheet that we copy and put in therapists' mailboxes after group (again, a template for the group email is available in Appendix A of this manual). Alternatively, individual therapists can gather this information in individual sessions when checking on other therapy modes.

Good News and Skills Group Check-In

DBT Next Steps group starts with two activities focused on mindfulness and contingency management. First, instead of a traditional mindfulness activity, group begins with each client and the group leaders reporting on good news from their week. The goal is to create the opportunity to receive positive reinforcement, to practice mindfulness of what is going well (or at least not wrong), and to start the group on a positive note to counteract any negative mood or thinking with which a client may have entered the session. This is a crucial social skill for clients to learn, particularly clients who have long gotten used to connecting with others through reporting what is going badly for them. For some clients, this also functions as exposure, as they may have a history of being invalidated when reporting good news and need the corrective information that most settings respond well to positivity and that it is a more effective path to receiving validation and support.

After good news all around, the group moves to the Next Steps Check-In. The Check-In practice is designed to help each client identify a long-term ambition (life worth living goals) that they are actually committed to achieving, learn how to identify Action Steps that are feasible yet challenging to work toward that ambition, and learn what effective and avoidant behaviors facilitate or get in the way of achieving Action Steps. For more details on the ambition and an example client ambition, see Appendix 3 of the *DBT Next Steps Skills Handouts* volume.

Each member of the group and the skills group leaders check in. Skills group leaders should follow a coping model—picking a goal that is within their personal limits to share that isn't too easy (you don't want your Action Steps to always succeed so you can model overcoming avoidance and problem solving) and isn't too hard (clients should get to see the leaders succeed). Often leaders will pick a goal related to a healthy lifestyle with Action Steps around exercise, relaxation, sleep, or diet, or something related to work that they avoid doing for mood-dependent reasons (e.g., timely documentation, timely response to an email).

The Check-In includes eight steps:

1. Stating your ambition (a.k.a. life worth living goals you are working on)
2. Stating the Action Step you committed to completing the previous week
3. Stating your progress on that Action Step (group practices providing reinforcement for progress that the client finds reinforcing)
4. Stating what was one effective behavior or thought that helped you with the Action Step
5. Stating one way you avoided if you didn't do all of your Action Step
6. Stating one way you will prevent this avoidance in the future
7. Describing one emotion experienced while working on the Action Step
8. Deciding on the Action Step to be worked on in the subsequent week

The group leaders and members are providing reinforcement for the ambition (Step 1) and progress (Step 3); help with validation, assessment, and problem solving of avoidance (Step 6); and planning the next Action Step (Step 8). Clients are encouraged to observe each other and "read the room" to determine if their attempts to reinforce are actually reinforcing and their suggestions are well received. Again, this provides practice for the many social interactions we hope clients are having outside of group.

The Check-In is part of the process of "learning to be your own therapist" or learning self-sufficiency. The Check-In treats many other problems, including:

- Addressing perfectionism, hopelessness, helplessness, willfulness, self-invalidation, and self-punishment in response to mistakes
- Directly targeting phobic avoidance of grand ambitions to teach clients to allow for possibilities
- Teaching clients to nonjudgmentally and openly self-observe their own effective and problematic behaviors so they can identify potential problems early—often before they even occur
- Teaching clients to effectively and quickly generate alternatives and to recognize small improvements so they do not jump ship before they can succeed
- Focusing on building upon success—choosing Action Steps that are the next logical steps and are sufficiently challenging to feel some pride of accomplishment (and get reinforcement from the group), yet not so challenging that they violate the shaping law that breeds success

After the good news mindfulness and the Check-In, the group moves to the review of assignments and, finally, to teaching the new material. A break can be taken at the end of Check-In, in the middle of assignment review, or before new material, depending on where a good midpoint falls. Given that the group session is 2 hours long, it can require careful time management when there are more than six members who need to describe both their Check-In and assignment. As with everything else, group leaders and clients are asked to be as effective with this approach as they would be in any work, school, club, or other time-limited meeting. Be prepared—have your good news ready, write out your Check-In on the worksheet provided, and write down your skills assignment so these all can be presented to the group efficiently. Group leaders should be prepared to teach the new material in as little as 20 minutes, if needed, and everyone should be able to work on using GIVE skills when steps need to be cut short or rushed.

Skills training for DBT Next Steps is the combination of new DBT skills with a more advanced group style that asks clients both to use their standard DBT skills to practice behaving in ways they need to in their new environments and to accept feedback when their skills aren't working. Capability to use skills is key to DBT Next Steps success and insufficient for most clients to overcome the approach–avoidance cycle caused by approaching feared situations. The next chapter focuses on how to overcome this with exposure.

CHAPTER 6

Exposure Strategies

Are Effective Behaviors Blocked by Problematic Shame or Fear?

Exposure strategies build one's capacity to confront a feared situation. After approaching a situation that has been previously avoided, exposure can create more balanced and realistic views of what is actually threatening paired with more balanced and nuanced physiological and emotional responses. In this way, exposure strategies lead to increased tolerance of fear and shame, rather than organizing one's life around avoiding feared situations.

The rationale for the huge role that exposure plays in DBT Next Steps speaks to the origins of how the treatment was developed. Many clients have very limited lives when they start SDBT (Linehan, 1993). Psychiatric disability or financial dependency often comes with a life that lacks obligations or consistent structured involvement in social, work, or school settings, and other life domains. As discussed in Chapter 1, for our clients who graduated from SDBT—free from the hospital and no longer in crisis—the new problem that emerged was that while these behaviors were gone or minimized, there were not enough QOL-enhancing behaviors developed to build a life worth living. Many clients continued in their financial dependency and/or psychiatric disability environment, perpetuating their fear, shame, misery, and quiet desperation. Shifting away from life-threatening and crisis-generating behaviors is a significant change, and that opens up a lot of unstructured time, with minimal demands and outside responsibilities to fill it. These clients can continue to languish in the dependency role. The social and financial rewards of working are absent, as is the general psychological benefit associated with meaningful work, active social connections, and a structured life. Also missing are the freedom and autonomy to make their own decisions, rather than the necessity to justify their decisions of where to live or how they spend their time and money to those who hold the purse strings. Many clients have clear work, school, and self-sufficiency goals, yet they simultaneously avoid Action Steps toward them, making these goals seem perpetually out of reach. To achieve their life worth living and shift the patterns of dependency, we recognized the need for developing a new approach that provided strong contingencies to create these new capabilities, block avoidance, and provide ongoing positive reinforcement for self-sufficient behavior within a treatment culture that prioritizes exposure to fear, frustration, and shame.

Exposure Is Integral to DBT Next Steps

Often, exposure starts in the first session of orienting to Next Steps, where hearing about the approach can elicit fear and shame. Continuing to discuss, assess, plan, and problem-solve in the face of action urges to avoid is key; however, this cannot be done in isolation without continuous positive reinforcement of the therapist. For example, if a client was fired from their last job, validating the fear they are likely to experience approaching a job interview is crucial, and so is simultaneously encouraging the client to attend the interview. Another dialectical approach to highlight the need for exposure could be the therapist entering the paradox by saying, "If you're not willing to experience fear, you'll be stuck with it."

The therapist takes the long view while validating the difficulty of the short view. Acting opposite to the emotional urge to flee (fear) or withdraw and hide (shame) is helpful in the long term to gain new learning about what's threatening, even if it is incredibly uncomfortable in the short term. Reinforcing steps toward approaching is essential, as the therapist uses many of the positive reinforcement strategies of contingency management in the effort to strengthen the client's progress in approaching new situations. Contingency management strategies are reviewed in Chapter 7.

The Role of Informal Exposure

Similar to SDBT, exposure strategies can be used informally or formally in DBT Next Steps. Informal exposure is used to reduce extreme emotional responses (e.g., fear, anger, guilt, or shame) and can also be used to suppress problematic avoidance or other behaviors. This is used frequently within treatment, and in some ways DBT Next Steps could be viewed as a shaping curve, increasing exposure and reinforcement of steps toward approaching more and more feared cues as the individual's life expands.

Informal exposure is also integrated into many DBT Next Steps skills and Recovery Goals related to emotional proficiency. Returning to the example of Janet (introduced in Chapter 3), a Recovery Goal that she consistently identified as being a priority was the ability to experience both positive and negative emotions building, staying, and falling mindfully, without avoiding them, rushing them along, or mentally moving into a different moment. The ability to do so—to increase informal exposure to emotional cues without suppressing or blocking—was related to many of her self-sufficiency and career development goals. For example, in order to regulate her interpersonal responses while interacting with dieticians and nutritionists as part of her career goals to become one, Janet had to work to regulate her emotional responses via exposure. This involved experiencing physical sensations of fear while observing urges to escape and not acting on them. Janet worked to regulate the primary emotional response of fear that would often be followed by a secondary emotional response of anger, creating problematic interactions with new colleagues. After a gradual increase in exposure to new social situations that activated a fear response, and building tolerance, Janet was able to integrate the corrective information into her awareness of what threat new social situations would realistically pose. She learned that her fear would spike and then subside relatively quickly after she mindfully observed the physical sensations and muscle tension. Reducing fear as a primary emotion proved to be an essential part of reducing anger as a secondary emotion. That is, once Janet integrated informal exposure to allow the primary response of fear to come and go more easily, she noticed a reduction in the anger and irritability that would historically be quick to follow.

To accomplish this, individual sessions focused on Janet strengthening several skills from the DBT Next Steps Applications of Mindfulness module that incorporate informal exposure strategies. Using the Mindfulness Skills for Anxiety helped Janet to understand that her avoidance behavior was limiting her brain from understanding that anxiety and related cues were not actually dangerous because anxiety was only spiking for lack of opportunities to observe it subsiding. Opening to What Your Emotion Has to Give You, the final skill of the module, offered Janet guidance for appreciating the functions of fear and shame to communicate the urgency of safety and belongingness. Rather than fearing the emotions, she began to practice acceptance and gratitude. The skill also provided steps and prompts toward observing the sensations and experiences of each emotional response as they would arise and subside. The instructions of this skill offered her an expanded framework to practice informal exposure, which she sought to build with the SDBT Mindfulness of Current Emotion skill, and was intermittently successful due to avoiding a fuller and in-depth intensity of practice. She would often "overthink it" and get lost in thoughts about the exercise that would take her out of the practice of observing physical sensations until the wave of the emotion could pass. The examples, metaphors, and more detailed instruction offered in the Opening to What Your Emotion Has to Give You skill seemed to resonate with her and foster willingness for more in-depth practice of allowing emotions to come and go. With the reduction in anger and irritability caused by the reduction in the primary emotion of fear, Janet had fewer action urges to criticize and lash out at others—expressions of anger that would often jeopardize relationships across all domains of her life. Informal exposure to fear and shame led to emotional freedom for Janet, allowing her to approach her career development activities with more ease.

In Vivo Exposure

In vivo exposure plays a central role in helping clients reach their Next Steps. Most clients' life worth living goals involve doing things they have never done or re-doing things that have gone terribly wrong in the past. Thus, their fear, shame, or frustration when approaching these activities makes complete sense. However, the clients underestimate one huge change: They have learned DBT skills that are incredibly useful in these situations. Being able to control one's attention with mindfulness, regulate one's emotions, tolerate distress, and be interpersonally skillful will serve the client well in such situations as working with an annoying boss, sitting through a boring class, meeting new people, forming a new romantic relationship, dealing with in-laws and family over the holidays, and the like. As such, the key DBT Next Steps strategy is exposure that, combined with DBT skills, succeeds to an amazing—sometimes awe-inspiring—degree. Often coaching required once someone is in these new environments is minimal and only needed for situations that we'd also be coaching our friends on and barely tolerating ourselves.

However, in the absence of sufficient exposure practice, clients remain too afraid, too humiliated from past failures, and too frustrated to face feared and frustrating situations, and it seems ridiculous to, on purpose, put themselves in situations where they failed in the past or where they believe they will be humiliated. Their reasonable mind may trust us when we say they have the skills and support they need to succeed; however, their emotional mind has only past experiences to go by and flatly refuses. In agreeing to move to Next Steps, they have to find Wise Mind to decide if they want to make the same commitment to do what those in exposure treatments for trauma have to do—commit to exposure in the service of their ultimate goals in order to learn the corrective information that things have changed, and they can now do things they could not before or have never tried.

In vivo exposure is going into the feared situations and staying there: mindfully looking all around, taking everything in, and fully participating in whatever needs to be done there. Such a strategy is not unique to this approach. Like social phobia exposure, *in vivo* exposure is about keeping one's attention squarely on what is happening in the moment and avoiding safety cues such as hiding one's face, doing ineffective preparation activities, or staying busy to avoid interaction. Processing how one appeared in the moment is saved for afterward or held for the therapy session to allow full participation while in the situation and to maximize the brain's opportunity for corrective information and habituation to fear, shame, and frustration.

In this perspective, it is critical to know "the facts on the ground," which makes a nonjudgmental stance and the effectiveness of Mindfulness skills critical. For example, if there is something the client doesn't know and needs to know to be eligible for a job, this cannot be overlooked because of mental self-criticism. By contrast, it is often the case that client's perfectionism or family pressure or invalidation has given them a distorted view of the standards the world holds them to, so full participation followed by mindful observation and description of the experience afterward offers the opportunity to learn that their performance was not only sufficient but also very good, or that the knowledge required was not nearly as high as they believed it was. Getting an entry-level job and being accepted into a community college are excellent examples of this. These are intended as settings for training and education, so they don't expect you to already have a great deal of knowledge going in. Some clients can aim much lower than their actual abilities, causing those potential employers or schools to see them as overqualified. It is only through *in vivo* exposure that the client—and their beliefs, physiological systems, and emotions—learn this to be true.

Since the DBT therapist is not a job coach in this model, they aren't physically present or helping the client. Instead, they are integrating exposure with other DBT strategies to increase motivation and capabilities. So contingency management—positive reinforcement for shaping adaptive behavior and blocking reinforcement for avoidance or retreat—is critical, as is assisting the client to understand what they experienced during the *in vivo* exposure. *In vivo* exposure may be a participatory mindfulness exercise the client does for homework, and then something they process in the subsequent session or out-of-session coaching.

It is also important to consider graded exposure (i.e., shaping the client's exposure to the feared cue through successive approximations, such as sessions of looking at pictures and then videos of elevators before sessions of visiting a building with an elevator, riding an elevator to the second floor, riding to the fifth floor, etc.) versus flooding (i.e., fully immersing yourself in the feared cue, such as getting into an elevator and staying in it and riding it up and down continuously until the fear subsides). Sometimes the client's situation dictates the answer. For instance, going away to college is inherently flooding—there isn't a reasonable way to shape into it. Similarly, moving out of one's home or moving to a new city is flooding. On the other hand, we generally require clients who are working to do so only 10 hours/week to start, and within that context, there are a lot of ways to provide more graded exposure options, such as volunteer opportunities or unpaid internships. For instance, a client whose career ambition was to be a landscaper/designer and needed to do their Work as Therapy chose to find a part-time job in the garden department at a big box home improvement store. This gave him substantial exposure to working with the public around gardening and helped him realize what part of that worked for him and what didn't. The income also allowed him to purchase a used car that was critical to carrying his landscaping gear to one-off and small garden jobs he was able to pick up. As he became more comfortable financially and emotionally and was more mobile, he added on a landscape design program through the community college to provide needed skills. By this time, he was doing garden-related work close to full time, having his emotions and physiology habituated and his beliefs about what is and isn't possible more accurate and nuanced.

Graded *in vivo* exposure also occurs through the process of reading about career options; writing a résumé; joining professional organizations or relevant clubs; applying for jobs, schools, sports teams, or clubs; building to interviewing; regular participation at a club or church; dating; then regular participation as an employee, student, member with good standing; or developing a romantic partnership. Recognizing the *in vivo* exposure nature of each of these steps and approaching them with that perspective (rather than just as problem solving and follow-through on agreed tasks) makes a substantial difference in what is being tracked on a Diary Card, the individual therapy discussions of what they did or didn't avoid, and the meaning of the client's fear in the therapeutic process.

The Role of Imaginal Exposure

In treatments focused on past trauma, imaginal exposure plays a central role, and *in vivo* exposure is used only strategically. By contrast, the focus in DBT Next Steps is on the future and, as such, *in vivo* exposure plays the larger role and imaginal exposure is used strategically but not centrally. Clients will have past trauma associated with the situations they have to approach to achieve their life worth living. In such cases, formal or informal imaginal exposure should be used, as in SDBT.

In addition, imaginal practice (such as in the Cope Ahead skill) plays a more central role. For clients who avoid situations when they need to approach, doing imaginal practice of approaching is a good use of individual therapy time. As in the Cope Ahead skill, first-person present-tense imaginal practice of going to a social gathering, job interview, financial aid office, and so forth is often employed to provide a graded exposure option. With the benefits of imaginal practice, the client and therapist can practice all going smoothly, all going wrong, and somewhere in between. This allows both habituation and an opportunity to problem-solve likely barriers. In-session or out-of-session coaching are opportunities to role-play feared situations with the therapist. Again, this provides both graded exposure and an opportunity to behaviorally assess where the client might go wrong and to practice cognitive restructuring of perfectionism.

In summary, exposure—particularly *in vivo* exposure—is a central strategy in DBT Next Steps. The model is based on our experience that fear, shame, and frustration are so dominant in the client's experience that these emotions are running the show. Some clients are experiencing this vividly as they wish so much to be changing their life. They are often swinging between the secondary targets of emotional vulnerability and self-invalidation when faced with cues of what they are missing—both of which are making things worse. Other clients are not experiencing any of these emotions because their avoidance behaviors kick in before emotions can make an appearance. In any case, there is no way through but to get started, lean in, partner with the DBT Next Steps therapist and/or group on the journey, and learn that most of what is dreaded is no longer true. All of which will be easier when the therapist is reinforcing strategically—the topic of the next chapter, contingency management.

CHAPTER 7

Contingency Management

Are Ineffective Behaviors Getting Reinforced?

Consequences follow behaviors, and the specific consequences can impact the likelihood of the behavior occurring again. For example, Janet submitted a round of job applications and shared with a friend that she was nervous about going for interviews. The friend shared that she was nervous on Janet's behalf, too—was now the right time to take on the stress of working when Janet almost had to go to the hospital last year? Janet had plans to follow up with all the employers she submitted job applications to earlier in the week, but after the conversation she talked in session about losing her motivation. She cancelled plans to spend time with friends and her church community, and she didn't check her email for the rest of the week, noticing a spike in shame, fear, and sadness with a flurry of hopeless thoughts. This example highlights the power of one's social network in influencing the likelihood of a client's behaviors occurring again in the future, particularly when they echo one's own self-invalidating thoughts and fears. The goal is to use the contingencies within DBT Next Steps to benefit the client in their self-sufficiency goals and provide a counterbalance to well-meaning but discouraging feedback from others. It takes quite a bit of mindfulness to figure out what the reinforcing consequences are and then rearrange them to follow the appropriate behavior. These techniques will be described in more detail after an initial review of the principles of operant conditioning.

Operant Conditioning Theory

Contingency management has its origins in operant conditioning theory and is used in treatment as the therapist highlights or reacts with specific consequences that either increase (reinforce) or suppress (punish) a client's behavior. To identify effective consequences, we must track backward in time to see what behaviors increased or decreased and then what happened right after that behavior. Positive reinforcement refers to adding something after a behavior that increases such behavior in the future, and negative reinforcement is taking away something after a behavior that increases such behavior in the future. For instance, love and attention after a teenager cuts themself can positively reinforce cutting. Negative emotions or experiences stopping, such as relief from anxiety or shame or someone removing demands after you cut, can be negatively reinforcing. By contrast, love and attention because it's a Sunday afternoon shopping date will positively reinforce many teenagers for normative teenage behavior. Using skills that provide relief will negatively reinforce skills practice instead of self-harm.

Positive and negative punishment works in a similar but reverse way. Positive punishment refers to adding something after a behavior that suppresses such behavior in the future and negative punishment is taking away something after a behavior that suppresses such behavior in the future. For instance, condemnation after cutting is likely to be positive punishment, and canceling the Sunday shopping trip because of cutting is likely negative punishment. However, suppressing a behavior has limited utility because it will re-appear in other situations when the source of the punisher is not present and tends to lead to avoidance of the source of the punisher. As avoidance of the therapist is not our goal, punishment has its limits in DBT. Table 7.1 provides a further overview of these ideas.

The timing and choice of positive and negative reinforcement are the core of contingency management. It is critical the therapist understands what each client finds reinforcing versus aversive, rather than assume it is the same as what they themself find reinforcing or what reinforces other people. For instance, some clients who have been starved for validation respond very well to effusive validation, whereas others are distinctly embarrassed by it and reinforced by much lower key reinforcement, such as offering a fist bump or brief eye contact and a smile and then moving on.

Reinforcing a problem behavior by maintaining eye contact and an engaged posture while telling the client not to do it sends a confusing message. Since nonverbal communication often takes precedence, this may result in reinforcement of, and therefore continuation of, the problem behavior. Therapists can practice in-session negative reinforcement (i.e., remove aversive consequences in response to adaptive behaviors) in response to this situation. The therapist

TABLE 7.1. Overview of Contingency Management Strategies and Principles of Operant Conditioning

	Increase behavior	Decrease behavior
Add consequence	*Positive reinforcement* Adding a consequence following an individual's behavior that increases the likelihood of such behavior occurring in the future	*Positive punishment* Adding a consequence following an individual's behavior that suppresses the likelihood of such behavior occurring in the future
Remove consequence	*Negative reinforcement* Removing a consequence following an individual's behavior that increases the likelihood of such behavior occurring in the future	*Negative punishment* Removing a consequence following an individual's behavior that suppresses the likelihood of such behavior occurring in the future

Note. From Carmel et al. (2016).

might withdraw attention by looking less directly at the camera during a telehealth session or showing less responsive and engaged body posture in response to the client rehearsing ineffective behaviors in session (e.g., fighting reality, blaming, or otherwise judging the problem at hand). This disengagement (essentially planned ignoring) is generally unpleasant for clients, so stopping it and bringing back eye contact and engaged posture as soon as the client constructively engages in problem solving often functions as negative reinforcement. The obvious downside of negative reinforcement is the need to add something aversive in order to remove it when the behavior becomes more adaptive. That is why catching the patient being adaptive and providing positive reinforcement are the most effective approaches.

Contingency management can be used informally in session during therapist–client interactions or more formally to create plans to increase relevant behaviors for the client. For a detailed but accessible introduction to contingency management, we recommend reading *Don't Shoot the Dog* by Karen Pryor (2018). For a detailed understanding of how to effectively observe and respond with maximal effectiveness to client's adaptive and maladaptive behaviors within the therapy session, we recommend reading *Functional Analytic Psychotherapy* by Mavis Tsai and colleagues (2012). Related resources for learning about reinforcement are also provided in the DBT Next Steps module on Perfectionism versus Reinforcement (see Chapter 15 and handouts in the companion volume, *DBT Next Steps Skills Handouts*).

Determining Behaviors to Increase

As discussed, positive reinforcement is adding consequences the client finds rewarding in response to adaptive behaviors in order to increase them. Positive reinforcement is the primary strategy used by DBT therapists to effect behavior change. It takes a lot of mindful assessment to figure out which behaviors are worth strengthening and which are worth weakening. To guide this decision, the therapist must consider how the behavior contributes to (or takes away from) each client's life worth living and Recovery Goals.

For example, Lee, who is working toward getting a raise and promotion, might work with his therapist to increase desirable consequences when he is on time for his work shift. On the flip side, in order to reduce lateness, Lee and his therapist might use contingency management strategies to remove the reinforcers that are part of the activities related to his lateness. This could include installing an app on his phone to block access to social media until a certain time of the day, so it is no longer available for Lee to access until after his shift.

DBT Next Steps therapists also look to communication with individual and group therapists as an opportunity for clients to practice interpersonal effectiveness and exposure, offering preparation and practice for entering new settings. For instance, a client is often coached to validate (without necessarily agreeing with) their DBT Next Steps therapist's perspective even when they adamantly disagree with it. What is ultimately needed for the client to thrive is the ability to generalize perspective taking and finding validity in a vastly different point of view from their romantic partner, professor, or manager in a work setting. Validation of the person holding a differing point of view (a real dialectic) might not be required for a client who has a career goal of becoming a park ranger in the wilderness, but if the client hopes to become a teacher, clinician, or fill another social role that requires flexible and responsive communication, they must demonstrate the ability to validate a different perspective in order to thrive.

Lee's therapist noted that the ability to find validity in an opposing position is key to working as a guidance counselor and supporting students who might have a different approach to navigating their personal and academic goals. Given that this was Lee's career goal, the therapist linked the target of validating a differing point of view to the goal of thriving as a guidance counselor. Linking the target to the goal fostered willingness and collaboration to remove the reinforcers that were part of the activities related to Lee's lateness, and to more actively validate the therapist's perspective.

Contingency management often involves shifting the reinforcers around so that they follow the behaviors we want to increase, rather than following behaviors we would like to suppress. Therapists must use a lot of nonjudgmental observing and describing to pull this off. Both therapist and client are on the lookout for the positive reinforcers for the client, asking the question "What consequences do they respond to?" (e.g., they talk more rather than less, their affect brightens up rather than getting more quiet and withdrawn). They must also ask, "Are the reinforcers lined up with a behavior we are working to increase, or does the reinforcer follow a behavior we are working to decrease?"

Determining the Reinforcers

As part of assessing what is actually reinforcing for the client, the DBT therapist observes their own communication style and considers its effects on the client. For instance, therapist praise following a completed assignment might be highly reinforcing and desirable to one client, but the next client might respond to praise as aversive: They might withdraw, become quiet, look away, or share dismissive or self-invalidating statements of their skills practice.

To understand patterns of reinforcement, it is helpful to look through a phenomenologically empathic lens. For instance, there are often legitimate and understandable reasons for a client to experience praise as an aversive consequence based on their learning history. The therapist's assessment can determine if this is the case, either through discussion with the client or observation of the client's behavior in response to different therapist actions. Perhaps, in the situation above, the client associates praise with new demands (e.g., "If I'm told I'm doing well, then I will be asked to do something new and maybe I won't be able to do it"), withdrawal of support (e.g., "If I can do it myself, others stop helping me"), fear of future disappointment (e.g., "If my therapist thinks I'm doing homework well, I'm bound to disappoint them with how I do on the next assignment"), or increased expectations (e.g., "Just because I did it today, they think I can always do it"). These examples, rooted in the biosocial theory of emotion dysregulation in transaction with an invalidating environment, generally occur without awareness and explain how some clients can experience praise as aversive. It also might explain how "active passivity" behaviors are maintained in the client's lives—problem solving and demonstrating efficacy at a task can actually lead to negative outcomes.

The praise example also shows how the therapist can't assume anything and must let go of assumptions about basic reinforcers that work for everyone. The therapist is wise to also consider why a response is aversive to a client, and to take note of these clinical data to build their case formulation. For instance, if the client withdraws and looks away after receiving praise from their therapist, are they likely to react in a similar fashion when their manager highlights an accomplishment at work? The therapist might hypothesize about the environmental origins and learning history, and work to find validity in the client's response based on their life experiences and conditioning (i.e., V-4 level validation—validation based on the individual's learning history or biology). While finding validity in the client's response is important, the therapist must also consider how the behavior causes problems and limits their pursuit of goals. A negative reaction to praise, such as disputing it or self-invalidating, might shape the client's manager out of giving them praise in the future. Absence of praise by a manager could also potentially lead to being overlooked for other common reinforcers such as raises, promotions, bonuses, or establishing seniority.

Therapist responses that are often reinforcing to a broad range of clients include acknowledgment of effort. Rather than praising the finished outcome of a high-quality assignment (e.g., "Excellent job with this!"), the therapist might have better luck validating the process of completing the assignment (e.g., "It must have taken a lot of skills to approach this homework and stay with it") or the effort involved (e.g., "I appreciate how much work you put into this").

Do the Reinforcers Follow a Behavior That You Are Working to Increase?

DBT Next Steps pays particular attention to providing reinforcers contingent on behaviors that indicate clinical progress (applying for jobs, taking steps toward a Recovery Goal), thereby reinforcing adaptive behavior change. Another example of the need to ensure the reinforcing nature of a therapist response occurs with skills-coaching procedures. For the client who is motivated to have additional contact with their therapist, it may be useful to create a contingency management plan whereby texts, voicemails, or general contact with the therapist are provided in response to the client exhibiting specific adaptive behaviors. For example, after submitting a job application, the client could text the therapist, who then responds with a high-five meme. The contingency plan would consider how the therapist's response could be reinforcing the client asking for help. The therapist could be clear they expect multiple attempts to be skillful or preparation for being skillful, like writing out a DEAR MAN script, prior to requesting coaching, so reinforcement of contact with the therapist follows skillful behavior rather than avoidance.

Let's return to Lee's target of increasing timeliness in order to advance and be considered for a raise and promotions at work. It's worth assessing the contingencies for timeliness and what happens instead of walking into work on time at the beginning of his shift. The therapist assesses the behavior and works to understand the consequence. What is so desirable about the activity that he's engaging in while he's supposed to be at work? Is the activity he's engaging in providing a consequence that is more powerful than being on time? Keeping an open mind and thinking outside the box are key here—often the reinforcing nature of a behavior is difficult to pinpoint and can be the least obvious to the therapist (or the client). For example, Lee sitting in the parking lot and communicating with a friend on social media when his work shift is starting might offer strong positive reinforcers. Communicating on social media might bring a sense of connection, closeness, joy, and humor to the moment. In this way, it functions as a positive reinforcer. However, sitting in the parking lot when one's shift is starting might also come with a sense of dread, stress, guilt, or other negative emotional responses. Entering in the communication on social media with their friend might be taking away these unpleasant experiences for some time, meaning this behavior might also be negatively reinforced: The moments on social media are moments when dread, stress, and guilt tend to subside. Alternatively, arriving at work a few minutes early might be the most effective behavior for Lee, but it might also be a time when he doesn't have a plan of what to do and a time when small talk is typical, both of which are anxiety-provoking. Lee might be in the parking lot waiting until the last possible moment, distracting himself with social media, causing him to lose track of time and arrive late. In such a situation, Lee could arrive early, prepared with GIVE skills to use with coworkers in the few minutes before opening, and his therapist and/or skills group could reinforce the use of GIVE skills. This will likely also result in natural reinforcements from his manager and other employees, both for being on time and for the relationship-building small talk. Thus, the contingency management within DBT is the bridge to reinforcement in the world that will maintain and generalize the behavior.

When the therapist and client have some idea of what the reinforcers are for the client, the next question is whether the reinforcers are actually following a behavior the client wants to increase (in this case, timeliness), as opposed to a behavior that the client is working to decrease (lateness). Stimulus control might be another thing to consider: Posting to social media might be an adaptive behavior to create positive emotions before walking into work, but it would need to occur earlier to prevent lateness. Helping clients to observe what the therapist is observing and use that information to become more skillful is asking a lot when clients enter SDBT with high emotion dysregulation, low mindfulness, and low distress tolerance. SDBT therapists often observe and adapt their contingency management to shape skillful behavior with little more than a highlight of the patterns they observe. By the time clients reach DBT Next Steps, though, they are not trying to get basic control and skills do not require as much active thought, so they are more able to learn to observe the contingencies in their life and to be their own therapist and respond effectively to maladaptive reinforcers.

Here is a different example. If clients are four or more assignments behind in Next Steps group, they go on suspension from skills group until they've got fewer than four back assignments due (as described in Chapter 5). Being out of the group is an aversive consequence that clients will work to avoid, similar to the four-miss rule and 24-hour rules in SDBT, which are other forms of negative punishment. However, unlike the four-miss or 24-hour rule where the withdrawal of therapy is for a fixed period, the duration of the suspension for back homework due is under the control of the individual. This brings in a reinforcement aspect, as with the "therapy vacation" in SDBT. Clients are welcomed back to therapy as soon as they've caught up on assignments, so the aversive consequence is removed as negative reinforcement for the client's action. As soon as the client has completed enough homework to be less than four assignments behind, they can rejoin the group, although the co-leader will offer coaching to get completely caught up as well. The leaders and group members will all be glad to see the client back and will share that verbally and nonverbally, which will be additional positive reinforcement for getting the work done.

"Contingencies create capabilities" is a motto we have in DBT. Lee will be capable of doing more adaptive things when contingencies reinforce them—that is, when there are positive consequences that follow a behavior to strengthen the likelihood it will occur again in the future or significant negative consequences for avoidance. It's a whole lot easier to finish tasks on a deadline or to clean the kitchen when guests are coming over. This is the key to orienting clients to the use of contingencies in DBT—contingencies are part of DBT because they allow us to make changing our behavior easier and thus make it easier to achieve our goals (for further discussion of this topic, see also Carmel et al., 2016).

Informal Contingency Management in Individual Therapy Sessions

Informal contingency management is primarily focused on reinforcing new and adaptive behaviors. The therapist needs to be sure they have the right reinforcers for the client and applies them whenever desired but rare adaptive behaviors occur. Over time, more and more adaptive behaviors appear and with ongoing reinforcement in the session and suggestions for out-of-session practice, these behaviors will occur in the world and also be reinforced there. Through the process of shaping, as an adaptive behavior becomes established, the therapist backs off to intermittent reinforcement of that behavior while continuously reinforcing behaviors that are new or appear inconsistently until they are also established. Given that the world around the client may not be systematically reinforcing their skillfulness, it is critical that the therapist and skills group leaders are doing so and teaching the client to recognize the process. This allows the client to get in on the act and start reinforcing themself and others, which, in turn, leads to more natural reinforcement.

The therapist should respond (or not respond) to maladaptive behaviors with the goal of reducing their frequency. Positive reinforcement is always the first approach. However, if a desired behavior is not occurring, shaping a smaller behavior should be considered. However, if the behavior is very important and shaping is not working, aversive contingencies or punishment can be considered. Punishment, as described above and in Table 7.1, is introducing a consequence following the maladaptive behavior that the individual will work to avoid. Punishment does not and should not imply being damaging or cruel. For example, if Lee begins consistently talking about reaching out to a dealer, the therapist might apply an aversive consequence. As this behavior is ineffective and found to be incompatible with the primary goals of self-sufficiency and keeping his job, the therapist might express disappointment or exasperation or directly confront the dysfunctional behavior. Use of aversive contingencies (i.e., punishment) should be used sparingly and mindfully, with a quick return to positive reinforcement once the client demonstrates a successive approximation of the effective behavior. The withdrawal of the aversive consequence then functions as negative reinforcement—the removal of an aversive experience. A therapist would quickly move from disappointment back to a stance of validation and warmth once Lee begins engaging in more "change talk" toward his recovery and discussing the negative impact of a relapse. It's key here to note that the therapist's aversive contingencies of exasperation and disappointment are directed toward the problem behavior of using and not the individual. In DBT Next Steps, just as in SDBT, the therapist strives to view their client nonjudgmentally and to communicate constant belief in them.

It is critical that the therapist be clear on what the adaptive behaviors are and describe them precisely. For instance, some clients complain a lot while engaging in very skillful behaviors or express hopelessness during behavioral rehearsal in session. It is critical to reinforce the adaptive behavior (being skillful) and ignore as much as possible other maladaptive behaviors that might accompany it (complaining, expressing hopelessness). Reinforcement is most powerful close to the desired behavior, so reinforcing progress and ignoring negativity as it occurs are often critical to promote adaptive behaviors in session. At a later point in the session, the negativity can be highlighted as a problem for the client to keep in mind or could be directly targeted with a chain and solution analysis.

It is easy for the therapist to miss the adaptive part of a behavior and get pulled in by the maladaptive part of a behavior. For instance, when a client says to a therapist, "What the hell do you want from me?," there is a problematic tone and cursing (maladaptive). However, the client is also expressing a desire to understand what the therapist wants from them (adaptive). We automatically respond to the nonverbal maladaptive tone and language over verbal communication so the therapist may well miss the adaptive piece. Even more likely, this is what will happen in a patient's life outside of therapy. So, it is important for the DBT Next Steps therapist to reinforce the adaptive part of the communication and teach the client to understand this whole process so they can see it and change it in their life.

It is also important to consider regional and cultural differences. For example, putting oneself down could be a problem for the client as it makes other people in their subculture embarrassed or at a loss for how to respond, but it could also be normative and considered self-deprecating humor. This comes up in DBT Next Steps when clients are moving into new vocational or social environments that may be like or unlike their own subculture, or like or unlike their therapist's subculture. This can lead to misunderstandings. It is important not to inadvertently punish culturally adaptive behavior. Therapists need to listen and assess for the response in the client's environment as well as their own response, and might highlight differences with the client in a culturally humble fashion that encourages an open discussion. The goal is for the therapist to understand exactly what behaviors are needed and will be reinforced in the client's environment, and the client has the opportunity to consider these cultural dynamics and contextualize their behavior without feeling judged. To meet this goal, the therapist must engage in therapy with the intention of honoring their client's unique beliefs, customs, and values. For instance, if a client reports making a joke to a friend that implies criticism of their friend's parent or at a business meeting that implies criticism of their boss, is this a problem? In some environments, not at all—people tease or joke about each other's failings all the time. In other environments, this could be considered unkind or unprofessional. In DBT Next Steps, we emphasize helping the client "read the room"—observe and describe for themself how others react verbally and nonverbally in response to what they say and do. It is important for the therapist to do the same.

Selecting and Applying Formal Contingency Management Plans

In addition to informal contingency management, explicit formal contingency management strategies can be used and taught to the client. The therapist, often in collaboration with the client, comes up with a "formal contingency management plan" to introduce reinforcers following effective behavior (i.e., rather than following the ineffective behavior). For example, Lee's therapist might pitch that, together, they create a formal contingency plan whereby Lee finds other reinforcers to get him to work on time, such as receiving a cheerleading text from the therapist right after he enters the building on time, saving a delicious snack or candy bar for right when the shift starts, observing the reaction of his manager or coworkers to his early or on time arrival, noting a sense of competency or confidence that emerges from tackling the difficult behavior of arriving on time, or observing the satisfaction that emerges from taking a step forward toward self-sufficiency. Several of these ideas were practiced by Lee, but shifting the most powerful reinforcer ultimately led to a change in behavior. When Lee (with his therapist's encouragement) chose to restrict social media until he went on break at work, rather than using the apps before work, he began arriving to work on time. The timing of when to allow a reinforcing consequence was key here, rather than finding a reinforcing consequence to match the power of social media, which proved to be quite difficult.

Ideally, formal contingency management plans will be based primarily on positive reinforcement, but they may include negative reinforcement, as necessary. Therapy does not generally involve a lot of aversives that the therapist has the power to remove. No one wants to be adding an aversive in order to remove it when the adaptive behavior occurs unless absolutely no effective behavior can be reinforced. So generally, positive reinforcement is easier and more effective than negative.

As people are complicated with rich learning histories, behavioral assessment is critical before moving forward with the best approach. Here are some examples to consider when troubleshooting your contingency management in DBT Next Steps:

- If the effective behavior appears, but not often enough, one can increase positive reinforcement whenever the desired behavior occurs while assuring no aversive consequences are occurring after the desired behavior. If Lee's manager and coworkers have kind facial expressions and say things in an upbeat manner when he arrives on time and not when he doesn't, this will provide reinforcement for arriving on time, which should increase its frequency. However, this will require Lee to make eye contact and mindfully observe their responses for him to be aware of the reinforcers. It will also require Lee to not add aversive consequences when he arrives on time, by invalidating himself for being late on other days or having thoughts that he's pathetic, to be pleased by their positive response.

- If the effective behavior has never occurred before despite the therapist teaching and practicing the behavior with the client and their commitment to do so, then shaping is likely needed. What is a component of the desired behavior the individual can do, and how can just that part be reinforced? In this case, the addition of arbitrary reinforcers, like Lee getting a favorite treat on the days he is on time for work, can get the behavior moving so Lee will experience his manager's approval, a natural reinforcer that will lead the behavior to continue.

- If an ineffective behavior is so dominant in how the individual responds to stress that no effective behaviors have a chance, then behavioral strategies like training an incompatible behavior are needed. In other words, the therapist could pick one feasible effective behavior that cannot occur at the same time as the ineffective behavior and train the client to do that. If Lee automatically responds to positive greetings when he is on time by saying something self-invalidating about his previous lateness, he could be trained to count to 2 or to 4 before speaking or respond with a hello + comment about the weather. The chances are the brief pause or time it takes to comment on the weather will lead to more skillful interpersonal behaviors and more positive responses from others, and will naturally start to replace the incompatible self-invalidating behavior. Training an incompatible behavior is a much better alternative to punishing the ineffective behavior.

In addition to the content of the formal contingency plan, the manner in which the therapist selects and implements the plan is key. A unilateral, "top-down" approach to planning, delivered forcefully with minimal responsiveness or collaboration on the part of the client, will naturally prompt defensiveness. It is important to recall the intended effect of increasing motivation for effective behaviors and decreasing motivation for ineffective behaviors. Contingencies that motivate clients to engage in behaviors that jeopardize their ultimate goals are not in line with DBT. Contingencies create capabilities, and expanded capabilities create a life worth living. Much like coaching elite athletes, the client's move toward their ultimate goals is an effort grounded in compassion and hope, even if getting there involves experiencing pain, vulnerability, and discomfort.

Figure 7.1 describes the three C's of contingency management: clarity, consistency, and collaboration (Carmel et al., 2016). These are considerations for how the therapist can select and apply formal contingency plans in a way that maximizes the chance of success. As the client moves into DBT Next Steps, the individual therapist should pivot from just managing contingencies to orienting and teaching the client about the contingencies at play in their life (see Chapter 8), collaborating with clients on formal contingency planning for therapy, teaching clients how to set their own contingencies to promote a better life, and generalizing this skill.

Contingency management offers a key opportunity for modeling by the therapist. Offering examples of how the therapist organizes the contingencies in their own life to promote skillful behavior can not only be instructive for the client, but also validate how normative it is to have these struggles. Modeling contingency management can take the following forms on the part of the therapist:

1. Identify situations in which the therapist is deliberately (or has inadvertently but successfully) set up contingencies that promote behavior that serves the therapist—for example, tying a walk for exercise with a phone call with a friend, resulting in walking being reinforced by the social experience instead of punished by boredom or fatigue.

2. If the therapist isn't aware of cases where they have done this, they should do so deliberately and observe the results. For example, the therapist can identify an ineffective behavior

Clarity

Clarity in contingency management plans requires that the client be adequately oriented. For example, during pretreatment sessions, clients are given the rationale for a plan and are asked to agree to it as part of treatment. Didactic strategies are used to teach behavioral principles and the effects of contingencies on behavior. The therapist provides transparency about the plans and why they are being considered. The DBT consultation team helps the therapist clarify contingencies operating in therapy and in the client's life, and to identify the behaviors, reinforcers, and aversives while selecting formal contingency plans and implementing them over time.

Consistency

Consistency is necessary to ensure that a behavioral plan will be effective over time. This often requires consultation from the DBT consultation team to address therapist and therapy-interfering behaviors, particularly a therapist's urges to avoid or deviate from a plan. The therapist uses a mindful approach to highlight patterns of behavior related to a plan to prevent inconsistencies from occurring and to problem-solve when inconsistencies have occurred.

Collaboration

A collaborative agreement is necessary to set a plan and to troubleshoot what could get in the way of implementing a plan. Consulting the client's Wise Mind on the reasonableness of a plan and its intended effect on obtaining their goals is key. Therapists will attend to the relationship and use commitment strategies to collaborate on a plan. For example, a therapist may ask, "How are we going to tackle this DBT Next Steps Work as Therapy requirement? We are 2 months away from the deadline and it's important that we come up with a plan now, so we don't have to worry about suspension later." Phone coaching can be used to help create a collaborative alliance around implementing a plan.

FIGURE 7.1. The three C's: Considerations for selecting and applying formal contingency management plans.

that is being reinforced, identify an incompatible behavior that is more effective, and change the contingencies surrounding the behavior until the effective behavior replaces the ineffective behavior.

3. It is important to orient to the concept of the "extinction burst"—a sudden spike in the frequency of a behavior when the reinforcement for that behavior is removed—and model overcoming it. The therapist could share how this concept has played out in their life while starting to change their own behaviors, or how they've responded to extinction bursts when setting contingency plans with others. For example, the therapist could share on the process of starting a contingency plan during dog training, and how their dog began barking even more when they first began removing reinforcers of barking. Keeping to the contingency plan and staying the course led to the dog barking less and less, even if that behavior initially increased. It's worth orienting to the principle of extinction bursts using similar examples given how often this shows up while changing long-standing patterns of behavior and developing new ones.

4. If necessary, bring the issue to the DBT consultation team. Team members can describe examples they have seen of how the therapist has managed their own behavior with contingencies or can help the therapist set up a practice scenario and stay with it until they have successfully shaped their own behavior with contingencies.

Regardless of the approach, the therapist now has examples to share with the client, and it will reinforce for the therapist how effective contingency management can be.

Normative Productive Activities, Career Activities, and Work as Therapy Contingencies

In the DBT Next Steps approach, three formal graduated contingencies are recommended to facilitate meaningful living wage employment: "Normative Productive Activities," "Career Activities," and "Work as Therapy." As introduced in Chapter 2, expectations of normative and productive behavior should be established as incompatible with the out-of-control behaviors targeted in SDBT. Until the client can organize their behavior around long-term goals instead of being entirely mood-dependent, they are not ready for DBT Next Steps. To promote practice organizing behavior around long-term goals, setting up formal contingency management for Normative Productive Activities in SDBT is highly recommended. This might take the form of 10 hours a week of normative productive activity 4 months into standard DBT and 20 hours a week of normative productive activity by month 8. Alternatively, the client might be expected to do a normative and productive activity every day before noon or every day before they can do something reinforcing, like playing video games or watching a favorite television show.

Normative Productive Activities

Normative Productive Activities are managed by contingencies and promoted via other DBT strategies. The therapist should define the Normative Productive Activities precisely and behaviorally so it is clear when they do and do not occur. "Normative," as defined in DBT Next Steps, means acting like you don't have emotional problems around other people who are acting like they don't have emotional problems. "Productive" means they are done with planning and purpose. The "three S's" of Normative Productivity focus on the quality of the activities that are chosen to ensure that they are (1) Structured, (2) Scheduled, and (3) Social.

The therapist needs to understand what is reinforcing and aversive to the client to ensure that reinforcement follows the normative productive behavior and aversive consequences do not. When natural reinforcement will not occur in response to normative productive behavior in the client's environment, the therapist and client can engineer artificial or arbitrary reinforcers. The client could tell the therapist when they engage in the behavior so they can get immediate reinforcement via text or messaging, or the client could give themself a quarter every time they engage in the normative behavior and use the money to buy something that gives them joy. Clients should be able to engage in regularly scheduled normative productive behavior prior to moving to DBT Next Steps given the fear, shame, and frustration that are expected to occur when they put themselves in new work, school, or social situations. If they can't organize their behavior for long-term goals and block mood-dependent behavior in general, we don't want to set them up to fail in more difficult situations.

Career Activities

The second formal contingency program, Career Activities, is tied directly to the client's personal employment ambitions and reflects the most effective activities to achieve them. This can include paid employment and/or college, vocational training, internships, self-employment, and so forth. A client who would like a career in nursing will need both a college education and related work experience, perhaps as a medical assistant or hospital volunteer. A client who wants to find a job in retail management, by contrast, likely needs to focus on working their way up within the retail sector; classes in management may be helpful, but academic training is less important in this case. A client who wants to be an artist or writer will likely need a living wage job that pays the bills and health insurance while leaving sufficient time during the week to paint or write, as well as the time and skills to market their work. Thus, they need to be able to succeed in jobs—even those they don't particularly enjoy—that provide benefits for less than full-time work (certain state jobs and some companies offer this option). If it allows them the stability to do the art they really care about, their enjoyment of the job may matter less.

Career Activities are decided by a synthesis of the client and individual therapist's Wise Minds and must have a direct tie to the client's career ambitions (e.g., taking an interesting college class outside of their career area does not fall under Career Activities unless it is an expectation of their college degree program). The DBT consult team can assist in deciding what to include and exclude from Career Activities when the individual therapist–client dyad needs help.

In a comprehensive DBT-ACES program, clients are required to be engaged in Career Activities for 10 or more hours/week by month 4 of DBT-ACES, and for 20 or more hours/week by month 8. If they do not do so for 4 weeks in a row after the deadline, they are suspended from treatment until they do, at which point therapy is reinstated as quickly as possible. When integrating DBT Next Steps into DBT in a less formal way, we still recommend having hard deadlines by which a client needs to have logged a minimum number of hours doing Career Activities. In the absence of a high-potency negative consequence, avoidance continues to dominate; sessions become focused on what the client *hasn't* done and everyone gets frustrated as therapy drags on. Remember, "Contingencies create capabilities." Lack of consequences may be the primary controlling variable for the avoidance, so you aren't making it easier for the client to succeed by being more nurturing or flexible in this case.

Work as Therapy

The third DBT Next Steps contingency, Work as Therapy, is based on the goal to assist clients to become financially independent of psychiatric disability, the social service system, and family or friends' financial support. For any client, there will likely come a time when they lose a job, get laid off, move to a new city, or otherwise have to start over. When they have to do this without disability payments, it means quickly finding a job and maintaining it—hopefully in their career area, although perhaps not right away. So, the idea is for the client to find and maintain a job on the open market to ensure they have the skills to (1) find a job quickly and (2) keep a job when it is financially necessary even if they don't like it. This means choosing a job for which anyone can apply (i.e., not in a sheltered workshop or working for your grandmother in a job she wouldn't offer to anyone else).

The "Therapy" part of Work as Therapy is that it functions as *in vivo* exposure to both job hunting and employment, as well as exposure to all the social aspects of work and the contingency management built into workplaces (e.g., consequences for not being on time, not getting along with coworkers, asking too many questions). The goal is that clients are learning these Work as Therapy skills as part of DBT Next Steps, so if they have already demonstrated they can successfully work a competitive job for at least 10 hours for at least 6 months, they do not need to be asked to do so again. Deciding if the client has these skills down is a decision for the client and therapist to make in consultation with the DBT team.

In a comprehensive DBT-ACES program, the Work as Therapy contingency requires finding a standard job on the open market and working there for a minimum of 10 hours/week for at least 6 months starting on or before month 4 of a 1-year program. As the skills learned in Work as Therapy are critical to any career, Work as Therapy hours count toward Career Activities hours. As noted above, by DBT-ACES month 4, the client is expected to be doing 10 hours a week of Career Activities. That means the client who is doing 10 hours of Work as Therapy is also meeting their Career Activities requirement. Work as Therapy hours, however, do not increase while, as specified above, Career Activities hours go from 10 hours at 4 months to 20 hours at 8 months. This is deliberate, to allow clients time to work on other Career Activities as appropriate to their life worth living goals like going to school or doing an unpaid internship. If their Work as Therapy job is the best path toward their career, then they can meet the Career Activities hours by increasing their work hours to 20.

If a client is not able to meet a formal contingency (i.e., Normative Productive Activities, Career Activities, or Work as Therapy requirement) for 4 consecutive weeks, they are suspended from treatment until they can achieve the contingency for 1 week using the principles of a "therapy vacation" in SDBT (i.e., do not offer DBT treatment, yet pine for their return, and coach only on how to return to therapy). To avoid unnecessary debate, the deadline to start suspension is always the first DBT Next Steps skills session of the week that contains the deadline, and individual therapy is restarted as fast as possible once the contingency is met—the day of, if possible. During suspension, the individual therapist does not provide therapy sessions and the client does not attend DBT Next Steps skills training. Coaching is limited to clarification of how the client can meet the contingency and cheerleading their progress. Crisis management is generally not needed, as life-threatening behaviors have stopped prior to DBT Next Steps; however, referral to other treatment can be made if necessary. If medication management is provided as part of the larger program, this continues, and the limits of the prescriber are reflected in how long they will see the client without concurrent psychotherapy. This also applies for continued enrollment in the larger clinic, if any. In our Harborview program, agency policy is that after 1 month of DBT-ACES suspension (i.e., no treatment other than medication management and pining for their return), we terminate the client's case. We provide informed consent, plenty of notice, outreach to prevent this occurrence, pining during suspension, and referrals for alternative treatment to avoid abandonment of the client. Assuming there are no issues with insurance coverage for treatment and the individual therapist is still available, the client is re-admitted immediately once they have met the contingency. If real-world issues like insurance interfere, the goal is to have the client back in DBT Next Steps immediately after they are resolved. Other clinics will have different limits and challenges following through with termination after a month of suspension. In lieu of termination, it is encouraged that, at minimum, the client be transferred to a non-DBT program within the clinic, since allowing for a return to the same DBT team without the client demonstrating the behavior would weaken these contingencies.

Several implications of the Career Activities and Work as Therapy contingencies are worth discussing. While most clients end up working more than the 10-hour minimum for Work as Therapy and it is usually easier to find work for 20 or more hours than for only 10, we selected 10 hours as the minimum for Work as Therapy to leave time for nonwork Career Activities such as school or an unpaid internship. We have learned that 10 hours/week for 6 months is enough of a behavioral sample to assess and resolve problems with working. Given that many clients have physical limitations, other responsibilities such as children or elderly parents, or limited transportation, we try to keep our requirements to a maximum of 20 hours/week throughout treatment. While this does not always work out in practice, the goal is not to exhaust or overwhelm the clients. On the other hand, if the client does not work many hours per week, the reduction in disability supports, such as housing or food stipends, will offset much of the earned income. Clients need to work enough hours per week that the amount earned relative to the amount of disability supports lost is big enough to be worth the effort. In our experience in the United States, this has meant working at least 20 hours a week.

Career Activities make inherent sense to clients pursuing Next Steps and are generally easy to define. Work as Therapy, on the other hand, requires substantial orientation and justification to clients as it is generally less obviously beneficial, less fun, more frightening, and the kind of activity in which they have previously failed and that led to disability in the first place. SDBT therapists can use commitment strategies in these discussions and link employment targets to a client's life worth living goals, while simultaneously validating the fear, frustration, and shame that would be expected for anyone as they approach goals where they had historically been unsuccessful. Clients are also encouraged to use the money earned at Work as Therapy to support their other Career Activities, such as buying a car or art supplies or paying for classes. We recommend that SDBT therapists begin orienting to these contingencies about 6 months before Next Steps so the clients have a chance to think about the implications and come to a Wise Mind decision about whether this is a challenge they want to accept. We find that even those who are sure they want to do it at first have commitment that waxes and wanes, and those who are at first unwilling often become more willing with time. Ideally,

SDBT therapists *want* their clients to move to DBT Next Steps, but do not *need* them to, so they can both help the client push forward while allowing them to make this big Wise Mind choice about their future.

Work as Therapy is not designed to be a poorly paid or otherwise negative job experience, which many SDBT clients think of when this is described to them. Occasionally, it begins that way, but most clients are able to find work in an area of general if not specific career interest (e.g., working in a pet store if they want to be a veterinary tech). In fact, it is generally easier to obtain a higher-paying job in an area of knowledge than it is to find many entry-level jobs they would hate. For example, working in a fast-food environment is what many clients presume we mean, but this is a challenging job that requires substantial mindfulness and distress tolerance skills to work at the required pace. We have found jobs for which the client has qualifications from their previous employment (e.g., working the information desk at a hospital or recycling center at a college) or that are related to their hobbies or life experience (e.g., landscape gardening at a city park, working at a child care center or doggie day care), where the employer pays equally well or better, offers benefits, or the client will enjoy the work.

Jobs in the client's career area may not be easy to get after a long period of unemployment but are more feasible from another job—such as a recent client who had medical assistant training, but could not get a medical assistant job. To meet the Work as Therapy deadline, she took a fast-food job while continuing to apply for medical assistant positions. Several months later, she got a medical assistant job, which she attributed not only to having a job while applying for it, but also the capacity to be on time, stick it out, be flexible, and so on, which she gained from the fast-food job. Both the fast-food and medical assistant job counted for Work as Therapy.

It is important for individual therapists and their clients to understand the implications of Work as Therapy on insurance and disability payments so they can problem-solve and troubleshoot effectively. In the United States, Social Security includes incentives to work, including a 9-month "trial period" of working above a specified level before the cash payment is withdrawn; however, Medicare insurance can continue long after disability payments have stopped. Clients can consult with social services or disability case managers to allow them to keep their disability even when they are working to meet this treatment requirement. In other situations, it makes sense for clients to investigate other health insurance options to pay for care before moving forward, so they are prepared if their coverage disappears when they work. In any case, this is a critical topic for many dialectical discussions and Wise Mind during SDBT.

The economy is also a necessary consideration when approaching Work as Therapy. The 2008 Great Recession in the United States brought into sharper focus the process of finding and maintaining work in the larger scope of Work as Therapy. If the deadline arrives and the client is not yet employed, there is often a question as to whether this is a result of the client's insufficient effort or the economy. To find a synthesis, we have developed a gradually increasing requirement of job hunting over the first 4 months of DBT Next Steps that has resolved this issue. Specifically, Work as Therapy now offers the following:

- If the client is already working a standard competitive job of their choice for enough time, they do not have to meet Finding a Job requirements unless they lose the job.
- Individual therapy focuses on the DBT Next Steps skills needed to look for, apply for, interview for, and accept a Work as Therapy job.
- Clients are free to use employment or other vocational rehabilitation services, but these

services are often very slow. This delay does not qualify for an exception to DBT contingency deadlines.

- Clients are required to submit an increasing number of applications once they start on Finding a Job until a job is acquired:
  Month 1: 1 application/week
  Month 2: 5 applications/week
  Month 3: 10 applications/week
  Month 4: 15 applications/week
- Given that often hundreds of online applications are submitted per job, online applications should not be the only applications completed. Clients should also look for work through their friends and social network, visit job sites in person, volunteer, and take other steps necessary to find work.

If a client has completed all of the finding-work steps, including this level of job hunting, without acquiring a job, then an extension of 1 or 2 months can be provided to the client's Work as Therapy deadline as long as they maintain 15 applications/week. However, a comprehensive DBT-ACES program is designed to occur concurrently with working, so if the client has still not obtained a job by month 6, they should be placed on suspension to ensure that the remaining 6 months of DBT-ACES occur at the same time as their work. It is our experience that DBT-ACES provided while a client is thinking about but not actually working results in graduates who continue to think about working without actually working. That is, working has to start while the client is in treatment and the therapist has time to help and troubleshoot until the client is comfortable working or they are unlikely to work after treatment. At least half of DBT-ACES provided to clients who are working results in graduates who continue to work. If using DBT Next Step strategies outside of a comprehensive DBT-ACES program, the individual therapist and team should consider these issues and decide how contingencies will be most effective in their program (see Chapter 11 for more on this topic).

In conclusion, contingency management in DBT Next Steps requires centering oneself around the DBT assumption that "clarity, precision, and compassion are of the utmost importance in DBT." The therapist must learn to see and define the behaviors of their clients in relation to the people and situations they are in—what drives what; what follows what. We have described the informal as well as formal use of contingencies as well as clinical examples to help therapists understand effective contingency management strategies. Reinforcement of adaptive behavior and remembering that "contingencies create capabilities" always come first. In the next chapter, we will consider how to use cognitive strategies to clarify these contingencies and overcome thoughts that inhibit progress.

CHAPTER 8

Cognitive Modification

When Beliefs Interfere with Building a Life Worth Living

Problematic thought content is likely to increase with new expectations for the client. The accountability, consistency, and self-reliance needed to succeed in work and school settings can easily prompt negative beliefs, underlying assumptions, and automatic thoughts related to the client's intense fear and shame. Cognitive modification addresses the problem of faulty, distorted, or incomplete interpretations. This approach has two primary procedures in DBT: contingency clarification and cognitive restructuring.

Contingency Clarification: "When You Do *X*, Then *Y* Happens"

The therapist uses contingency clarification to help the client notice and extract contingencies operating in their life. Observing the contingencies at play is helpful before working to change employment, school, or self-sufficiency. Highlighting the behaviors and their related consequences can be an important first step before working toward behavior change. The use of "contingency clarification" is key here; it means letting the client know that when they do *X*, then *Y* occurs. The therapist works to help the client recognize patterns and increase awareness and insight.

For example, as discussed in Chapter 7, the therapist targeting Lee's lateness at work discovered that he was in the parking lot on his social media app when he was supposed to start his shift. Contingency clarification might take multiple forms with this scenario. The therapist could highlight to Lee that being on social media likely has strong positive reinforcers (connection, humor) and negative reinforcers (taking away dread, stress, and guilt about work). The therapist might work to clarify contingencies by nonjudgmentally describing them, such as

"When you are on Snapchat in the parking lot when your shift is scheduled to start, it appears to bring connection in a moment when you feel disconnected and filled with fear, dread, and urges to avoid. We would call this the positive reinforcement of Snapchat. At the same time, have you noticed that, while you are on the app, the dread you feel about your work shift tends to decrease? I think being on the app also takes an uncomfortable emotion away—we'd think of that as a negative reinforcer." The therapist had previously clarified the contingencies of other behaviors and their positive and negative reinforcers for Lee, including his drug use that was a high-priority treatment target. Lee's cocaine use brought positive reinforcers of feelings of euphoria and negative reinforcers of taking away judgmental self-talk and low mood, at least temporarily. For Lee, observing the range of reinforcers and working to replace them with more adaptive ones were essential parts of becoming sober.

Aside from acknowledging the emotion regulatory consequence of the behavior, the therapist might just as easily clarify other consequences. When Lee is late, it could easily communicate disrespect to his manager and coworkers, and send the message that neither the job nor their time is valued.

With contingency clarification, the therapist must let go of assumptions. One client might possess knowledge of the social effects of their behavior and an understanding of how social, work, or school environments respond to the behavior of lateness. Another client might need to build this awareness; their lack of awareness could account for why they are not meeting expectations. Case formulation can provide a framework for understanding these struggles. The biosocial theory of emotion dysregulation suggests that there are relatively less presence and engagement in one's environment when the client is doing well and the environment is more responsive during emotional escalation (Linehan, 1993). Neglectful home environments are often characterized by the child receiving less observation and feedback in general. This environment can create a deficit in self-reflection and awareness that we seek to address in therapy with increasing mindfulness of the effects of one's behavior, in this case via contingency clarification.

The therapist is communicating the rules that are operating in new work or social situations that the client is entering into and noting the appropriate expectations. Lee, for example, might be surprised that his lateness has a negative effect on others, particularly in work settings that are new to him. Work settings functioned quite differently from Lee's home and social settings where lateness was largely the norm. Tolerating others' lateness with minimal reaction was also the norm. Embarrassment and shame spiked after his therapist pointed out the consequences of lateness as potentially communicating disrespect to his coworkers. This was met with encouragement from the therapist and validation about his reactions based on his learning history and social norms (V-4 level validation). At the same time, the therapist actively targeted this skills deficit by increasing more awareness of the norms of the work culture he was currently part of. For Lee, whose Career Plan focused on working as a guidance counselor, he began becoming more mindful of the social norms of his current job at an academic advising office and how they differed from the more casual and collaborative environment he encountered as a volunteer at a youth drop-in center. Lateness among volunteers at the drop-in center was common and tolerated. The norms of the academic advising office were to arrive on time and work more independently. At his job in the advising office, Lee focused on the Mindfulness of Others skill and working to generally "read the room." Rather than just clarifying contingencies of ineffective behavior, the therapist is wise to also use the strategy to shape effective behavior. This proved useful as a positive reinforcer once Lee began changing his behavior and noticed he was receiving better responses at work. He would also experience pride and joy when his therapist clarified the positive contingencies; that is, Lee's timeliness prompted praise by his manager and opened up opportunities for seniority with scheduling and a promotion.

Cognitive Restructuring: Flexing the Rigid Interpretations

Cognitive restructuring offers a set of tools to replace rigid or distorted interpretations with more balanced ways of thinking. Cognitive restructuring is part of a range of CBT strategies that are considered the hallmark of behavior change; however, this approach in DBT is more explicitly dialectical in nature than in CBT. We are working to consider what is being left out.

Consider Janet's experience starting retail work and encountering difficult interactions with customers with multiple needs and demands. This was also a huge increase in social interaction compared to what she was used to given the years of isolation she endured before getting the job. She wasn't used to communicating with many people, particularly in the role of point-person with others who needed information from her. Her beliefs and assumptions about other people had limited flexibility since she had very few opportunities to test them prior to working retail. With the encouragement of her therapist, Janet identified thinking patterns and assumptions that customers disliked her. With specific customers, she worked to consider the evidence to support that notion and a different notion as well. With cognitive restructuring, we are seeking another perspective; adding another side to reduce the polarization that comes with rigid and inflexible thinking. For example, let's look at the interpretations that prompted anger for Janet during her work shift. It's possible the customer disliked something else about the store, such as the music playing rather than Janet, or maybe they got little sleep the night before and were grumpy in general. Check the Facts is a primary skill in SDBT to work to increase flexible thinking; however, cognitive restructuring procedures can borrow from a large set of established, empirically supported CBT tools to increase adaptive thinking (e.g., Socratic method, thought records, downward arrow).

Applying cognitive restructuring involves first assessing what the problematic beliefs, assumptions, and thoughts are that are inflexible, rigid, or judgmental and lead to problematic emotional responses, action urges, and subsequent actions. It's similar to contingency clarification and other change procedures: Mindfulness to identify what is problematic is the first step before changing things.

In DBT Next Steps, it is important to consider the styles of thinking given the goals of self-sufficiency. Several cognitive distortions are usually "par for the course," given what is likely to happen for people when they start approaching new environments, increasing expectations, and questioning their role in their "dependency environment." Common cognitive distortions include catastrophizing (exaggerating the significance of an incident), overgeneralizing (seeing one incident as part of a global pattern), or personalizing (believing that incidents are caused by you or are about you). Orienting to the likelihood of these thought patterns arising can be a helpful way of preventing future problems during an interview or midterm exam.

The DBT Next Steps therapist may consider which thought patterns are present when the client is first oriented to the program. It's important to take a "thought inventory" and assess which cognitive distortions are likely to arise. They are likely to arise again and again when new environments are approached and the client's life expands. Mindfulness of thinking styles helps the therapist and client be ahead of the game. They expect these beliefs and assumptions to arise, rather than being surprised when they prompt emotions and problematic action urges.

Janet's catastrophizing following a difficult interaction when she was irritable with a customer led her to believe that she would get fired. Ultimately, this incident did not even make it onto her next performance evaluation. Rather, she was given more responsibility after that evaluation. The therapist highlighted that the outcome ran counter to the belief she held that getting fired was inevitable due to the incident with the customer. Cognitive restructuring involves highlighting when there is evidence to support an alternative assumption. The idea is to increase dialectics: The therapist might encourage the client to observe and describe their situation mindfully. This involves encouraging the client to "take in" both their initial interpretations as well as an alternative interpretation to flex their beliefs, rather than discounting the evidence and continuing with a rigid and fatalistic interpretation.

As these examples illustrate, many clients come into DBT with hopeless thoughts about achieving real change in their life and have many rationalizations for their avoidance behavior. These beliefs and expectancies can hold them back from the *in vivo* exposure they need to make big changes. They can also support the incorrect idea that contingencies are a problem rather than a help in achieving their goals. Thus, DBT Next Steps individual and group therapists need to be vigilant for problematic thoughts and expectancies, and move in to help the client observe the dialectic and find a synthesis. Knowledge is power—and this goes beyond understanding your own problematic behavior to understand how behavior works in general and the typical ways that it goes wrong. This is the focus of the next chapter on didactic strategies.

CHAPTER 9

Didactic Strategies

Teaching as Well as Doing

In DBT Next Steps, the didactic strategies play a major role as we frequently teach the clients what we are doing in DBT rather than just doing it. We want to teach clients to be their own therapist so we are much more likely to explicitly teach them what we are doing and how they can do it too. As noted in Chapter 8, contingency clarification is teaching clients the ifs–thens of life and therapy. This helps the client make sense of different environments and their own reactions: observing and describing what is going on so the client can decide how to respond, be it with acceptance or change.

Linehan (1993) describes didactic strategies in SDBT as follows:

> The essence of the didactic strategies is the imparting of information about factors known to influence behavior in general, and of psychological, biological, and sociological theories that might cast light on particular behavior patterns. . . . Usually didactic information is imparted as it relates to effective methods of behavior change and self-control relevant to the patient's own problems. However, at times such information is also useful in understanding the behavior of others related to the patient. This didactic strategy is used to help the patient focus on relevant information during behavioral analysis, to generate solutions, and to make decisions and commitments to specific goals in treatment. Information given didactically is meant to counteract overly moralistic, superstitious, and unrealistic views of behavior and change. The assumption is that patients with BPD are often woefully lacking in such knowledge; they frequently have inadequate information about factors that typically influence behavior and about normative responses to situations in which they find themselves. This lack may be due to a variety of factors, including the deficient or faulty teaching and learning typical of invalidating environments. (pp. 272–273)

In SDBT, the didactic strategies play a critical role in orienting the client to DBT, including teaching the diagnosis of BPD, the biosocial theory, and the principles and elements of chain analysis. However, time is precious and TIB is frequent in SDBT, so it is optimal but often infeasible to give session time to teaching explicitly what the therapist is doing. In addition, clients who are behaviorally out of control and overwhelmed by their emotions are often not in a position to care about why or how DBT works. Thus, we generally get on with using the strategies and only occasionally highlight why we are doing them.

DBT Next Steps is in a different clinical situation altogether: The client is generally regulated and their behavior not out of control or in crisis. Instead, the client is stable yet stuck, trapped in old patterns and avoidance; unable to reach their ambitions because they cannot mobilize themself into new and challenging behaviors that serve their long-term goals. In this context, learning what is happening behind the curtain can be particularly useful in helping clients mobilize and motivate themselves for their long-term goals.

Over the years, and especially through the revision of the original SDBT skills manual (Linehan, 2025a, 2025b), Marsha Linehan incorporated more therapist strategies from DBT and other interventions into the skills taught to clients, including:

- Interpersonal Effectiveness Handout 6A: Expanding the V in GIVE—Levels of Validation
- Emotion Regulation Handout 8: Check the Facts
- Emotion Regulation Handout 12: Problem Solving
- Distress Tolerance Handout 17: Dialectical Abstinence
- Distress Tolerance Handout 19: Community Reinforcement

In the DBT Next Steps Skills Curriculum, we have continued this approach. We have included skills based on therapy interventions that can be found in Part IV of this manual and in the companion skills-training manual for clients, including:

- Perfectionism and Reinforcement Week 3: The Basics of Reinforcement
- Perfectionism and Reinforcement Week 4: Untraining or Making It Stop!
- Succeeding after DBT Week 2: Therapy-Interfering Behavior
- Mindfulness Week 3: Using the Mindfulness Skills for Anxiety

Didactics about DBT strategies and therapeutic strategies from other interventions are routinely discussed in individual DBT Next Steps sessions as they arise and are relevant to the client's targets and goals. Teaching about and also using DBT strategies demands clarity, precision, and compassion. If the therapist is not deliberately using a DBT strategy (e.g., exposure, systematic reinforcement of adaptive behavior), it will be difficult to explain and demonstrate its relevance to the client. This is sometimes the root of problems that therapists have as they move down the DBT hierarchy from life-threatening behavior and nonattendance and noncompliance TIBs to QOL-interfering behaviors and noncollaborative TIBs. The therapist is not yet competent at DBT themself, so targeting less concrete behaviors is more challenging. In such cases, it is recommended that the therapist—preferably with their DBT consultation team—go back to the DBT manual and take time to read and discuss elements of DBT that they don't fully understand, and to figure out how to reinforce themself and each other to be competent at these strategies. This is an excellent reason to seek supervision or peer consultation from a DBT expert.

Once the therapist is clear about the DBT strategies, the choice of when to prioritize the didactic strategies versus just doing DBT becomes the question. Step back and consider whether the behavior is pervasive enough that it affects multiple DBT targets. The absence of sufficient positive reinforcers for taking risks is an excellent example that is common when a client has a history of trying new things and quitting in a crisis or who has loved ones or care managers who are especially protective. We have treated many clients for whom we are the only people in their lives championing them as they make big changes. In such cases, teaching patients the principles of reinforcement can be very helpful prior to problem solving. Their understanding of why they are doing what they are doing and how they are affected by those around them often leads to greater acceptance of the need to expand their world to new people who will reinforce new things. For example, a client who attends an Alcoholics Anonymous meeting where unemployment or underemployment is the norm may change to one where the norm is being employed and self-sufficient. Thus, they are more likely to receive support for finding and keeping work than avoiding it. This change might be a smaller and more doable first step than applying for jobs, while providing the environment they need to naturally reinforce employment-related behavior. Understanding the principles of reinforcement can help the client make a variety of choices on their own rather than being dependent on the therapist to give specific advice.

TIBs are often good targets for teaching DBT strategies: Are comments from loved ones reinforcing avoidance of an Action Step to apply for school? Is the client's inability to validate in the moment making therapy tiresome for the therapist? Is rigid thinking the reason the client is resisting looking for work? Is the client losing commitment in the face of hard challenges? Many of these situations lend themselves well to teaching the client about the DBT strategies we use as therapists, and how they can use them in their own lives. Linking in-session behavior to out-of-session behavior, we can help clients to see how DBT strategies and skills can make therapy better while also improving their QOL and helping them to achieve their goals.

In summary, didactic strategies are core to DBT. We try and give the client all the knowledge that will help them achieve their goals. The processes that guide behavior change become more explicit rather than implicit, more transparent rather than hidden, more collaborative rather than led solely by the therapist. The difference in DBT Next Steps is how often we make the DBT strategies themselves what we teach so clients can learn to be their own therapist.

CHAPTER 10

Smoothing the Process
Validation, Dialectics, and Commitment

There is little other than the content and process of therapy that is unique about validation, dialectics, or commitment as you move from SDBT to DBT Next Steps, so this is a shorter chapter. Having said that, applying validation, dialectics, or commitment strategies might look different given the changing circumstances that clients encounter as they move toward self-sufficiency and financial independence. This chapter includes several considerations for how to use these strategies in the nuanced targeting of Recovery Goals and other QOL-interfering behaviors.

Validation

As with SDBT, DBT Next Steps uses all levels of validation and emphasizes functional as well as verbal validation. As has been extensively discussed, discouragement is common in DBT Next Steps and must be both validated and counterbalanced with validation of the client's inherent and learned capabilities. Cheerleading—a core validation strategy in DBT—is highly emphasized in DBT Next Steps to both counterbalance discouragement and hopelessness in the session and to prevent it between sessions by helping the client observe, self-validate, and accept that they have what they need to succeed.

In SDBT, the therapist working with a behaviorally dyscontrolled and hopeless client is equated to "being the football coach of the lowest-rated high school team in the league during the final game of the season. The team is behind 92 to 0 in the fourth quarter; three people are left in the stands" (Linehan, 1993). By contrast, in DBT Next Steps, the therapist of the stable but stuck client is more like the coach of a team with the opportunity to go to regionals—then maybe nationals—for the first time. Nonetheless, the job is the same: "The coach . . . stands firm, shouts encouragement, and inspires the team to keep going. In short, the coach cheerleads" (Linehan, 1993).

As in SDBT, in Next Steps, the therapist uses all the cheerleading strategies including assuming the best, providing encouragement, focusing on the client's capabilities, contradicting/modulating external criticism, providing praise and reassurance, being realistic but dealing directly with fears of insincerity, and staying near (Linehan, 1993). It is obvious that all of these strategies will be critical when clients approach difficult tasks and things they have failed at before.

For example, when Janet experienced fear and dread about applying to a job, her clinician communicated belief in Janet's ability to apply for it and succeed. The clinician acknowledged Janet's fear and dread as an understandable reaction, and at the same time, Janet was asked to borrow some hope and confidence from her clinician for the time being until she was able to grow more hopeful and confident herself over time. Reviewing and consciously practicing the cheerleading strategies will help keep the wheels of progress well greased.

Dialectics

Janet's example above also illustrates the use of dialectics while encountering hopelessness, fear, and dread. When working in Next Steps, DBT therapists use all the dialectical principles and strategies as they would in SDBT. There is a greater likelihood that the therapist will teach dialectical strategies to clients (see Chapter 9) and encourage the client to take the lead in observing and describing dialectics in their environment, rather than telling clients what dialectics they see (at least not before the client gets a chance to try). DBT presumes that change is a natural life occurrence. Allowing natural change while focusing on QOL means allowing room for clients to encounter inconsistencies, consider new limits, and endure failures. These are all normative experiences for the person adjusting to a broader life, with a broader range of environments that have a broader range of expectations. The DBT Next Steps therapist is the "cheerleader" who will provide relentless validation to the client as they go through these various transitions. At the same time, the DBT Next Steps therapist is also the "drill sergeant" who pushes them forward toward a self-sufficient, financially independent life without giving way to extinction bursts or urges to give up or quit.

Commitment

Commitment is a crucial part of DBT Next Steps (for further discussion, see Chapter 13). There is really no hope of progress on any life worth living goals without the client's desire to go there. A therapist may have to accept that a client doesn't want to work or go to school or otherwise make big changes in their life (for all the reasons described in Chapter 1); however, building commitment, being devil's advocate, and strengthening commitment are all equally important in Next Steps.

For example, when Lee expressed urges to quit his volunteer work, his clinician responded by saying, "I'm open to the idea that now might not be the moment to continue volunteering. However, what if the moment actually is right now? This is the path forward that will lead to other paths for building the relationships and independence that you yearn for. It's up to you in your Wise Mind about whether you want to keep walking on the path. However one thing is for sure, you won't get to your destination as quickly if you don't keep going." This stance of "freedom to choose in the absence of alternatives" appealed to Lee's autonomy in making the decision while highlighting the consequence of not walking the walk of his commitment.

As with SDBT, it is important to be awake to loss of commitment and move in with commitment strategies when needed. On the other hand, DBT therapists remain aware that lack of action is often not about a loss of commitment. One can be very, very committed to lose weight or get in shape or study for a big exam and still procrastinate, avoid, and otherwise fail to do what is needed for success. Not presuming a loss of commitment or making an interpretation like self-sabotage is standard in DBT as well as DBT Next Steps. It is important to consider multiple controlling variables for the lack of needed action and match the treatment strategy to the problem at hand.

PART III

INTEGRATING DBT NEXT STEPS INTO A COMPREHENSIVE DBT-ACES PROGRAM

CHAPTER 11

The Structure and Logistics of DBT-ACES

As recounted in Chapter 1, DBT Next Steps was initially developed as a structured 1-year program to follow standard DBT called DBT–Accepting the Challenges of Employment and Self-Sufficiency (DBT-ACES). This model has been evaluated and shown substantial increases in employment and career goals in pre–post studies. However, over time, we have seen the value of particular strategies and approaches when used outside of a structured DBT-ACES program and the value of the DBT-ACES skills on their own. In Part II of this book, we presented these strategies and skills as Next Steps for moving clients not only away from their out-of-control behaviors but also to a life that will support their hopes and dreams. In Part III, we describe the comprehensive DBT-ACES model in this chapter, then the DBT-ACES pretreatment process that we believe is an intervention in itself (Chapter 12), and finally when and why a DBT team might choose to incorporate some DBT Next Steps strategies into an existing program, implement DBT Next Steps as a follow-up to SDBT, or implement a comprehensive DBT-ACES program (Chapter 13).

A comprehensive DBT-ACES program pulls all of the elements of DBT Next Steps together in a 12-month treatment that follows SDBT. These various components are listed in Table 11.1. Generally, as clients' out-of-control behavior subsides and the focus is moving into QOL-interfering behavior, the idea of DBT-ACES is introduced, particularly when there are big changes that the client wants to make that they are avoiding, have failed at before, or have a history of quitting. The pretreatment process for DBT-ACES (described in Chapter 12) generally takes a couple of months. Often, however, the idea of taking the leap to DBT-ACES means taking the leap to living wage employment, moving out of their parents' house, going to college, or other big changes, and it often takes clients a while or some considerable starting and stopping to get through pretreatment and into DBT-ACES. DBT-ACES pretreatment includes having a career plan and a résumé, which can take time to develop. In addition, it is easier to meet the Work as Therapy and Career Activities contingencies if the client has started meeting

TABLE 11.1. Summary Descriptions of Unique DBT Next Steps Strategies

DBT-ACES Recovery Goals

DBT-ACES is guided by a set of specific goals to increase behaviors that are needed to find and maintain employment as well as overall self-sufficiency. Recovery Goals include several quality-of-life domains that are tracked daily using a Diary Card and are reviewed quarterly in a client self-assessment to determine which areas need to be prioritized to achieve life worth living goals. The domains include Living Wage Employment and Off of Psychiatric Disability, Interpersonal Proficiency, Emotional Proficiency, Life Outside of Work, and Self-Management.

Normative Productivity Requirement

Normative functioning is defined as acting as if you don't have mental health or emotional problems around others who are acting as if they don't have mental health or emotional problems. This normative functioning occurs in a "productive" manner by being structured and scheduled outside of the client's home. The aim of this requirement is to increase exposure to new settings and expand opportunities for social connection, or at least enter into new environments where social connection is more likely to occur, while working to decrease depression and anxiety that are often associated with social isolation, unstructured time, and limited demands outside of the home.

Work as Therapy Requirement

Work as Therapy is a graduated contingency to facilitate becoming financially independent of psychiatric disability, the social service system, and family or friends' financial support. To ensure that clients have the skills to find a job quickly and keep it until they find a better one, the Work as Therapy contingency requires finding a standard job on the open market and working there for a minimum of 10 hours/week for at least 6 months.

Career Activities Requirement

Career Activities is a graduated contingency to facilitate living wage employment in a desired career. These hours are directly tied to the client's career ambitions, which often are not the job they are currently working as part of the Work as Therapy requirement. Specific activities are determined by the client and individual therapist and include college, internship or volunteering in their desired field, self-employment, etc.

DBT Next Steps Check-In Practice

During the Check-In section of DBT Next Steps groups, every client and co-leader remind the group of their long-term ambition and then report on their progress on an Action Step toward that ambition, what they did that was effective to achieve it, any way they avoided working on it, and emotions they observed. The Check-In practice is designed to help clients to (1) identify a long-term ambition that they are committed to achieving; (2) learn how to create tangible Action Steps that are difficult, yet possible, to take action toward the ambition; and (3) observe the effective and avoidant behaviors and emotions that facilitate or get in the way of achieving Action Steps.

DBT Next Steps Skills Training

The DBT Next Steps skills curriculum includes the following modules: Perfectionism versus Reinforcement, Establishing and Re-Evaluating Relationships, Time Management, Managing Emotions Effectively, Succeeding after DBT, and Applications of Mindfulness. Skills-training topics address common problems for clients who are stuck or avoiding change, such as cognitive rigidity and perfectionism, inadvertent punishment of their own skillful behavior, poor management of time, and struggles interacting effectively with non-DBT clinicians. The goal is for clients to learn and then generalize these skills in work, social, and self-sufficiency contexts, as well as understand the specific steps needed to create their own social support system and effectively interact with new and established friends, people at work, and treatment providers.

the Normative Productivity contingency during SDBT and begun looking for work if they are not already working. Thus, we recommend starting DBT-ACES pretreatment (i.e., starting an application for a DBT-ACES program) 6 months in advance of when they would intend to begin DBT-ACES.

DBT-ACES formalizes the DBT Next Steps strategies into a unified program explicitly focused on living wage employment and self-sufficiency. Chapter 2 compared the elements of DBT Next Steps and SDBT, which applies to DBT-ACES as well. DBT-ACES individual therapy is structured by the Recovery Goals (Chapter 4), and a DBT-ACES version of the Diary Card is used to capture the client's daily progress. The four primary change strategies apply: skills training (Chapter 5), exposure (Chapter 6), contingency management (Chapter 7), and cognitive modification (Chapter 8). Didactic strategies (Chapter 9) are emphasized because teaching the client to be their own therapist is an explicit goal of DBT-ACES. We tell clients our goal is that by the end of DBT-ACES, they may *want* further therapy but won't *need* therapy to stay afloat and manage their emotions and behavior.

All three work contingencies are implemented: Normative Productive Activities, Career Activities, and Work as Therapy (Chapter 7). Based on the timing for a 1-year DBT-ACES program, clients need to be working a minimum of 10 hours a week by the end of month 4 of DBT-ACES. While these 10 hours also count toward the Career Activities and Normative Productivity contingencies, Work as Therapy often dominates in the early period of DBT-ACES. By 8 months into DBT-ACES, clients need to be spending 20 hours a week on Career Activities. This could be met by working 20 hours a week on Work as Therapy or could be met (all 20 hours or some part of them) with school, a training program, unpaid internship, self-employment, or relevant volunteer work. This moves the focus to the client's desired career in the second half of DBT-ACES and hopefully sets them on a strong road to living wage employment in their chosen profession.

DBT-ACES clients attend a 2-hour weekly skills group using the DBT Next Steps curriculum (see Part IV of this book and the handouts in the companion book for clients, *DBT Next Steps Skills Handouts*), including starting with Good News, then the Check-In, Assignment Review, and New Material. The curriculum takes 6 months to complete, with six modules taught one module per month. Thus, in a 1-year DBT-ACES program, the material is taught twice. As with SDBT, there are advantages to a second trip through the skills in terms of increased practice and the ability to better integrate the skills the second time when the other Next Steps skills are already in their repertoire. However, like SDBT, there are reasons why a DBT-ACES program might be 6 months with only one trip through the skills. For instance, adolescents and young adults who have recently spent a lot of time in a learning environment often can pick up skills very quickly and have fewer years of ineffective behavior to unlearn. DBT-ACES offered in a short period could be an effective way to jump-start them back into the Next Steps of their peers such as college, apprenticeships, or entry-level employment. While DBT-ACES can be completed in 6 months, the work contingencies need to be sped up to ensure that the client is getting a considerable amount of time in DBT-ACES while employed to receive the maximum benefit.

The DBT-ACES consultation team is generally just the DBT program consultation team rather than a separate team. Time is dedicated every quarter to a review of the Recovery Goals of each of the DBT-ACES clients through their self-assessment, which is part of skills-training homework quarterly. This is also reviewed by the individual therapist to be sure what the therapist thinks they are targeting matches what the client thinks, and any issues with which Recovery Goals should be targeted are discussed and debated among the team. As there are more Recovery Goals than a therapist–client dyad could treat in a year, figuring out which are the core issues that require therapy and in what order to address them is a place where the team can be of great help.

The consultation team also helps to support all members and to hold one another accountable while implementing the various DBT Next Steps contingencies. Therapists often need validation and problem solving from the team when their clients are unable to engage in the behavioral requirements of the DBT-ACES program. Table 11.2 reviews the timeline and duration of these requirements and the consequences that occur when they are not met, which generally involve the client going on a period of suspension from therapy ("therapy vacation" in SDBT) until they demonstrate the required behavior and are welcomed back. This is critical because DBT Next Steps works best when a substantive part of the treatment occurs simultaneously with work, school, social engagement, and building self-sufficiency, and we have not found that clients start these behaviors after DBT-ACES if they weren't already doing them during DBT-ACES.

Moving these work contingencies forward can sometimes prompt negative emotions for therapists and clients alike. Many therapists will struggle with urges to avoid taking these steps or find themselves on the side of "compassionate flexibility" about whether suspension is needed, when "unwavering centeredness" to go forward with consequences is what's actually needed. Thus, consulting with team members can validate the difficulty of upholding the behavioral contingencies of DBT-ACES, while ensuring that the necessary steps are taken to follow through with suspension. It's a team effort to stay the course of therapy suspension when DBT-ACES program requirements are not met and to maintain a clear, collaborative, and consistent approach to contingency management. Pining for the client's return by both the individual and group therapists is crucial here, as it is with any therapy vacation in DBT, to assure the client that their care has not been terminated and the therapist is confident they can do what is needed to return to treatment.

As noted above, DBT-ACES is explicitly time-limited to 6 or 12 months. The goal is to no longer be dependent on therapy or public mental health, so the DBT-ACES individual therapist pays particular attention to plans for after the client graduates from DBT-ACES. The Succeeding after DBT skills-training module (Chapter 19) helps to focus both the client and the therapist on what could hold the client back from leaving treatment altogether or resolving barriers to receiving high-quality care for circumscribed issues after DBT-ACES (e.g., Stage 2 or Stage 3 issues such as trauma care, treatment for a remaining disorder such as obsessive-compulsive disorder [OCD], or couple counseling). In addition, the DBT-ACES individual therapist will work with the client to consider who will be following them for psychiatric medications following DBT-ACES so this can be started early, as it is very difficult to find a prescriber comfortable with taking on a DBT patient as the sole provider at the end of DBT. However, we have found that if the client transitions to a new long-term prescriber fairly early in DBT-ACES (4–6 months into a DBT-ACES year), then the prescriber is comfortable taking them on and can observe their progress as they start work or school and see how the DBT-ACES therapist manages the client's distress through the process. Often, the prescriber will ask that in order to see them, the client will need to remain in therapy so they will not be the sole provider. However, as the client continues to improve despite taking on big challenges in DBT-ACES and demonstrates

TABLE 11.2. Contingencies, Time and Duration of Requirements, and Consequences in a 12-Month DBT-ACES Program

Contingency	Time and duration of requirement	Consequences if not met[a]
DBT-ACES-interfering behaviors: maintaining no life-threatening or serious therapy-interfering behaviors	Can only start DBT-ACES after 8 consecutive weeks without DBT-ACES-interfering behaviors occurring. Continue no DBT-ACES-interfering behaviors for the duration of treatment.	If DBT-ACES-interfering behaviors take place, client is placed on probation status and is suspended from treatment immediately if the behavior happens again. Client is then not eligible to return until they have 8 consecutive weeks without DBT-ACES-interfering behaviors.
Normative Productivity requirement	Throughout DBT-ACES, maintain 20 hours/week of normative/productive activity.	If there are 4 weeks of <20 hours, the client is suspended from therapy, during which time the only contact with team members is to coach the client to resolve the issue driving suspension and to pine for their return (Work as Therapy and Career Activities count as Normative Productive Activities).
Work as Therapy requirement	During the course of SDBT and/or DBT-ACES, clients are required to work 10 hours/week at a Work as Therapy job for 6 months. This job must start by the end of 4 months into DBT-ACES.	If there are 4 weeks of <10 hours after month 4[b] of DBT-ACES, the client is suspended from therapy, during which time the only contact with team members is to coach the client to resolve the issue driving suspension and to pine for their return.
Career Activities requirement	By the end of 4 months into DBT-ACES, maintain Career Development activities 10 hours per week. By the end of 8 months into DBT-ACES, maintain Career Development activities 20 hours/week.	If there are 4 weeks of <10 hours after month 4[b] of DBT-ACES, or <20 hours after month 8[b] of DBT-ACES, the client is suspended from therapy, during which time the only contact with team members is to coach the client to resolve the issue driving suspension and to pine for their return.
DBT-ACES skills group assignments	"Back Homework Due" in skills group: Clients must be no more than three assignments behind in group.	If clients are four or more assignments behind in group, they go on suspension from DBT-ACES until they've got less than four back assignments due, during which time the only contact with team members is to coach the client to resolve the issue driving suspension and to pine for their return.

[a]Given that treatment is not being provided during a DBT therapy suspension, after a prespecified period agreed upon with the larger program or agency (e.g., 4 weeks), the client may need to be discharged from the program. However, every effort should be made to re-enroll the client as soon as criteria are met.

[b]If DBT-ACES is conducted in less than 1 year, due dates should be shortened to ensure that at least half the treatment occurs while the client is working.

the ability to use skills and not exhibit out-of-control behavior or be in crisis, prescribers have sometimes decided they are comfortable continuing to prescribe without concurrent therapy, if the client requests it.

DBT-ACES means doing all of DBT Next Steps in a formal way focused on achieving major progress toward living wage employment in a career of the client's choice through an intensive, time-limited program. In the next chapter, we will describe the pretreatment process that sets up clients to succeed in DBT-ACES. Then, in Chapter 13, we will discuss the pros and cons of doing some or all of DBT Next Steps within existing DBT versus establishing a DBT-ACES program.

CHAPTER 12

DBT-ACES Pretreatment

Overview of DBT-ACES Pretreatment

Reflecting a comprehensive DBT-ACES program's focus on employment and college, pretreatment for DBT-ACES uses an application process that combines principles of a job application, performance evaluations, and a job interview with the self-reflective essays of college applications. This chapter explains the formal pretreatment process used in DBT-ACES, and in Chapter 13 we discuss how it applies to DBT Next Steps outside of a comprehensive DBT-ACES program.

The goal of pretreatment is to be sure not only that the client is committed to DBT-ACES but also that they are prepared for the challenges; it often serves as an intervention in its own right. The DBT-ACES pretreatment approach maximizes opportunities for exposure to unjustified fear, anger, and shame, and contingencies are set to create new capabilities for the individual. For those who come from SDBT in the same DBT program as DBT-ACES, pretreatment orientation begins 6 months into SDBT to ensure that the client has sufficient time to understand what is involved and consider whether it is in their Wise Mind to continue from SDBT into DBT-ACES, compared to other DBT and non-DBT options available to them. For those interested in coming to DBT-ACES from another SDBT program, there is no prescribed time frame, but as previously noted, pretreatment often takes clients 2 months to complete and is extended by client's avoiding the application, so we recommend starting several months ahead to understand and complete the process.

As with SDBT pretreatment, the goal is not to exclude clients but rather, as Marsha Linehan says, to "make it hard to get in and then accept everybody." We orient them to the differences between SDBT and DBT-ACES including potential barriers to success and the commitments they need to make. We use all the commitment strategies and follow initial commitment with a devil's advocate to build and troubleshoot commitment. The goal is for everyone to successfully complete pretreatment and enter DBT-ACES. Multiple tries are validated and reinforced as perseverance and determination. Clients can re-apply until they get in.

At the same time, DBT-ACES is an advanced DBT program, and we try to make DBT-ACES pretreatment an intervention that provides exceptional learning opportunities for those seeking a productive and satisfying life outside the disability/dependency/social service system, while minimizing the possibility of failure. In our experience, clients who have been successful in this have demonstrated competency in three areas: (1) competence with the SDBT skills, (2) ability to voice and demonstrate desire for a productive and satisfying life outside mental health and social services, and (3) minimal TIBs. DBT-ACES pretreatment is designed to build all three and we have found that it has been beneficial, even when someone ultimately decides not to complete the process and join DBT-ACES.

As noted above, DBT-ACES pretreatment is organized around an application process that blends typical work and college processes. Pretreatment has five steps, each of which provides the clients with an opportunity to demonstrate their skills in specific areas. The five steps of pretreatment are:

1. Written application completed by the client
2. Group leader and individual therapist performance evaluation of the client's behavior (with the client making a request to each for them to complete this)
3. Providing a résumé
4. Passing a test of SDBT skills competence
5. Completing an interview with the DBT clinical director or DBT-ACES group leader

The last two steps are completed after the application and other materials are submitted to the DBT-ACES consultation team for review. The pretreatment materials are available in full online at www.dbtnextsteps.com, and the DBT Next Steps Pretreatment Materials: Client Application and Individual and Group Therapist Performance Evaluation forms can be found in Appendix C of this book.

Some clients and SDBT therapists find the pretreatment process onerous and worry that it is a barrier to DBT-ACES. It can be a long process and demands a lot of initiative on the part of the client. A poll of DBT-ACES therapists, however, found that no one wanted to remove a section or shorten the application as each step was considered to be a useful intervention. Pretreatment—as with the program—requires accepting the challenges of employment and self-sufficiency. Psychiatric disability is extremely hard to leave and easy to return to. It is not realistic, in our opinion, to expect clients to be able to make these changes easily.

It is helpful for DBT-ACES pretreatment if the SDBT individual therapist has been framing QOL targets and targets on the Diary Card in ways that reflect the Recovery Goals, even before they are explicitly introduced to the client. With this groundwork laid, pretreatment serves to orient the client to what is needed to achieve the Recovery Goals using the DBT-ACES approach. As with SDBT pretreatment, the therapist uses a devil's advocate to encourage clients to voice or strengthen their reasons for making this commitment. DBT-ACES pretreatment also helps clients make a choice by highlighting the alternatives. If they would prefer an employment program that does not lead to living wage employment but works within the limits of the disability system or family financial support, there are standard vocational programs to assist with this, both within and outside the mental health system.

Clinically, we have found that it is important that a definitive decision about whether a client is leaving SDBT and entering DBT-ACES occurs at least a month before the client's SDBT contract period is scheduled to end. This is because a client might not complete all the pretreatment steps before the end of treatment. We do not want the therapist and client still working on the process right up to the end of SDBT treatment, giving them no time for closure or planning for the future. To facilitate this, the application and performance review steps are due one skills module before the end of the SDBT contract period, and the rest of the pretreatment steps must be done 1 month before the end of SDBT. If the client does not complete pretreatment by this time, they are welcome to continue to apply or take a break and apply at a later time, but the individual therapist will pivot away from a plan for DBT-ACES and move to therapy-ending strategies for the last 1–2 months.

If a client's Wise Mind is to take a break between SDBT and DBT-ACES, that is perfectly acceptable. This often happens when SDBT has brought them from the pit of hell to a place of no or limited pain and positive social connection. Sometimes the thing to do at that point is just relax and enjoy the accomplishment. Clients may want to return later because the status quo after SDBT becomes boring, or at a preplanned time, such as "I'm taking it easy this summer and will see you for DBT-ACES in the fall," or "I would like to do a trauma treatment first and then work on these big life changes afterward." Those who choose to take a break often complete most of the pretreatment steps before the end of SDBT, but they can also end SDBT and complete pretreatment later. The one issue that will require troubleshooting in this case is that once the client completes SDBT, they won't have the added assistance of a DBT provider through the pretreatment process, and the performance evaluation step needs to be flexed. The rest of this chapter will expand on the pretreatment steps, including adaptations to account for those completing the process without the support of a DBT provider.

Pretreatment Step 1: DBT-ACES Client Application

The DBT-ACES Client Application gives clients an opportunity to apply their DBT skills as well as the problem-solving and behavioral assessment strategies they learn in SDBT to their future choices. These skills are typical of graduates of SDBT programs but are often not explicit. As seen in the DBT Next Steps Client Application form provided in Appendix C, the application helps clients to observe and describe key issues with regard to a self-sufficient life, such as their Career Plans, Recovery Goals, and operant reinforcers of disability and dependency behaviors. In addition, the application provides an opportunity for clients to demonstrate that they can observe and describe relevant problem behaviors, thoughts, judgments, emotions, and TIBs, and mindfully and effectively respond to them. For each issue, the application functions as troubleshooting: What have they changed since coming to SDBT? What still needs to change for them to be ready to face a job and/or college? What commitments do they need to make in DBT-ACES? What could get in the way, and how will they resolve the issue?

The individual therapist provides coaching to strategize how to complete the application while expecting the clients to do the work themselves. Strategies to improve sections that are insufficient are discussed in session. Therapists continue to coach until a sufficiently complete application is prepared (this generally takes one or two drafts; occasionally more). We have found that giving the client the entire DBT-ACES application packet to review provides a needed overview, and yet clients should be encouraged to do only one section of the application at a time. Focusing attention on only one section and reviewing it in individual SDBT therapy help the client think through their choices, and this makes a huge difference in their readiness for DBT-ACES. Even if clients decide against attending DBT-ACES, the application can help them clarify their Next Steps in building a life worth living.

Sometimes, clients can become frustrated that the entire application focuses on how their behavior is an issue and not on external challenges, like difficult therapists or how life has made things hard. Issues such as these should be validated as absolutely correct. The application is an evaluation of their ability to describe and consider their piece of the puzzle and figure out how to overcome the limitations of others and the system. Why? Because most job applications, school entry criteria, and the like are also based solely on the applicant's capacity to do the work regardless of the workplace. Additionally, the ability to move forward in the face of an external problem is necessary to escape the many, many ways that the social and mental health systems inadvertently hold clients back. If the client needs their environment to be hospitable to achieve success, they will likely be blocked almost immediately in their process to return to work and exit social services. This is why DBT-ACES stands for Accepting the Challenges of Employment and Self-Sufficiency because it is a challenge that cannot be changed and must be accepted and overcome. Again, it is helpful to introduce the DBT-ACES concepts and application by month 6 or 7 of a 1-year SDBT program because clients need time to find dialectical synthesis on this for themselves and decide whether DBT-ACES is the challenge they want to pursue.

Pretreatment Step 2: Individual Therapist and Group Leader Performance Evaluations

In addition to their application, the client also needs to submit performance evaluations—completed by their individual therapist and a group leader—rating the frequency of specific client behaviors related to success in DBT-ACES as well as work, school, and other real-world environments. In order to succeed in employment and in the DBT-ACES program, clients will need to effectively manage their behavior and emotions in both boring and challenging one-on-one and group situations. The purpose of the performance evaluation is for the group leader and individual therapist to provide feedback to the clients highlighting their strengths as well as constructive feedback on areas where they can improve. These reflect the approach that clients need to perform in DBT-ACES therapy as they would on a job, in a college class, on a date, or with family and friends.

Performance evaluation forms (see Appendix C or the Resources page of www.dbtnextsteps.com) focus on the client "throwing themselves into DBT" by completing assignments, attending class on time, and effectively participating in class discussions and exercises. These ratings are scored in percentages or frequency of their occurrence in the past 2 months of treatment. In addition, there is a focus on the applicant's interpersonal interactions with others in group. Clients need to show that they are able to effectively manage interpersonal dilemmas, read and adapt to social cues, take direction productively, ignore others' dysfunctional behavior, and use interpersonal skills to obtain desired outcomes if they are about to enter the workforce. Also, if the client has or is currently having interpersonal struggles with another group member, they need to be willing to "turn the mind" to what is effective, use GIVE skills effectively when irritated, and give the benefit of the doubt to the other (stepping away from judgments), while staying emotionally regulated in spite of the stress. These are skills needed in the workplace and classroom, and basic competence in these areas is needed before entering DBT-ACES.

The performance evaluation forms use rating categories comparable to what is seen in typical workplace evaluations. This not only provides feedback about the client's readiness for Work as Therapy, but also provides exposure for clients who experience fear or shame when faced with a performance evaluation. Clinicians are asked to consider the client's behavior in each category over the past 8 weeks and designate the level that most accurately describes their performance.

- **O**—Outstanding. The candidate consistently exceeds expectations, requiring little or no coaching or feedback.
- **E**—Exceeds Expectations. Results clearly exceed expectations on a regular basis. Performance is of high quality and is achieved on a consistent basis.
- **M**—Meets Expectations. Competent and dependable performance level. Meets the performance standards and objectives without constant follow-up/direction, though intermittent coaching may be needed.
- **I**—Improvement Needed/Unsatisfactory. The candidate does not meet performance expectations on a regular basis and has difficulty following through with tasks. Requires regular and consistent follow-up and/or coaching.
- **N/A**—Not applicable or too soon to rate.

Clients must at least achieve Meets Expectations in the majority of items to be considered ready for DBT-ACES.

To provide maximal learning and minimal worry for the SDBT client, the DBT-ACES pretreatment materials also contain optional "interim performance evaluations" for both the individual therapist and the group leaders. The interim forms are shared only with the client to give them an idea of their standing prior to the pretreatment reference. Many clients like to give these forms out as soon as they start considering DBT-ACES in order to learn where they stand now, so they can improve any behavior that might show poorly in their final reference. For example, if DBT-ACES is introduced to the client 6 months into SDBT, the client might give the interim evaluations to their therapist and group leader then. Feedback from the interim evaluation can lead to improvements in group and individual therapy, so when they arrange for the pretreatment performance evaluations to be completed a few months later with their DBT-ACES application, the ratings of the previous 2 months don't include the earlier time when there were problems and allow the client to look their best. Interim evaluations are only for the client's benefit and are not required.

Pretreatment Step 3: Résumé

Once clients begin DBT-ACES, they have 4 months to find employment for at least 10 hours/week. This is a short time frame. While not required, individual therapists in SDBT generally have their clients seek work prior to the start of DBT-ACES to reduce the pressure of meeting this deadline. However, DBT-ACES applications do include a copy of the client's résumé. There is no particular format or guidelines for this because (1) the expected résumé format is different for a welder versus a nurse versus an artist and (2) résumé expectations change over time. As long as the résumé is appropriate to the field the client is pursuing, it is acceptable.

Assuring that the résumé is completed prior to DBT-ACES is necessary so that clients can immediately start applying to at least one job a week, as is mapped out in Work as Therapy (see

Chapter 7). We have also discovered that résumés are often something that triggers a lot of avoidance and over-editing that can take up a lot of time within DBT-ACES, so it's important to have it ready to go beforehand.

Pretreatment Step 4: Test of SDBT Skills Knowledge

After the team has reviewed the submitted application materials, including the performance evaluations and résumé, the client can then complete the final two steps of pretreatment. Knowledge of SDBT skills is evaluated by having the client complete and pass a written test, as well as through the exercises built into the DBT-ACES application. The purpose of the test is to assess the extent to which clients are able to describe, give examples of, and apply particular skills on demand. The questions on the test cover mindfulness, interpersonal effectiveness, emotion regulation, and distress tolerance skills. The exam is five pages long with questions presented in different forms, including multiple-choice, matching terms, short answer, and fill-in-the-blank. A score of 75% or greater is considered passing. Study materials and skills module quizzes to prepare for the exam are available to clients. It can be re-taken as many times as needed to pass. (Any test of all the DBT skills would be appropriate to use for this purpose, but materials for the test that we developed can be accessed on the Resources page of www.dbtnextsteps.com).

Pretreatment Step 5: DBT-ACES Interview

Once the application is completed and approved by the individual therapist, the client schedules a one-on-one meeting with the clinic director or a DBT-ACES group leader (or another DBT team member who is not their individual therapist and is preferably least known to the client) to present the materials and be interviewed about their readiness to begin DBT-ACES. This is a commitment session designed to reinforce the client's progress, orient to the ways DBT-ACES differs from SDBT, confirm the client is committed to DBT-ACES and strengthen that commitment, and troubleshoot potential problems. The exercise also functions as a behavioral rehearsal of interviewing and exposure to the thoughts and emotions that may arise.

The first question of the interview asks the client to describe their desired life in 5 years, assuming that DBT-ACES is effective and they achieve their goals. The client is expected to describe a life outside of financial dependency, with meaningful employment, adequate and satisfying social support, and positive self-image. If the client gives some but not all of such a story, the interviewer prompts the client (e.g., "And what about a romantic relationship—would you like that?" or "And how about your job—what would you like to be doing?"). We have found that the ability to answer this question with a picture of independence and normative functioning is very predictive of success in DBT-ACES. If the client paints a picture of minimal work or disabled living, the interviewer should challenge them to see if they can improve the image. If not, the client should be directed to discuss this further with their individual therapist. Often the client may not actually be interested in DBT-ACES but wants to continue with their individual therapist for another year or doesn't really understand what they are getting into. This provides the opportunity for the SDBT individual therapist to target such issues and help the client (and therapist) find Wise Mind.

Second, the interviewer challenges the client to provide assurances that life-threatening and self-harming behaviors have stopped and that they have "closed the door" to suicide and self-harm. The interviewer generally orients the client to the fact that DBT-ACES requires a lot of individual therapy time that won't work if the individual therapist needs to focus on life-threatening behaviors. The client is oriented that they will then likely fall farther and farther behind their compatriots in DBT-ACES skills group and find it harder to catch up. Thus, if self-harm or suicide risk is still an issue, the interviewer wants to protect the client's precious and limited time in DBT-ACES for when it can be of the most use to them and directs the client back to the individual therapist to resolve suicide and self-harm risk thoroughly prior to DBT-ACES enrollment.

If there is a question about the client's TIB in SDBT or other readiness for DBT-ACES, it should be identified in a DBT consultation team prior to the interview. Usually, the interviewer asks the client's therapist, "What should I focus on in the DBT-ACES interview?" TIB is targeted next in the interview, in the same way self-harm or suicide risk is addressed. If any life-threatening or TIB is not resolved, the interviewer takes the issue back to the DBT consultation team. The team may require that the client wait to enter DBT-ACES until the client can go 8 consecutive weeks without DBT-ACES-interfering behaviors occurring. Alternatively, if DBT-ACES-interfering behaviors have occurred recently enough to be of concern but not in the past 8 weeks, or have occurred in the last 8 weeks yet are unlikely to re-occur, the DBT consultation team can accept the client on probation. In that case, should the DBT-ACES-interfering behaviors re-occur, the client would go on immediate suspension until it is resolved for 8 consecutive weeks.

For example, an SDBT client had stopped self-injury by month 6 of SDBT, and in the weeks prior to the DBT-ACES final decision at month 11, he cut himself. The client would either be asked to wait to start DBT-ACES until 8 weeks of no cutting occurred or, if the client and therapist are sure this was a total aberration that is now solved and won't occur again, the client could enter DBT-ACES on probation, and would be suspended from treatment immediately if they cut again (until he had 8 consecutive weeks of no cutting).

Finally, the interviewer orients the client to what to expect practically and emotionally in DBT-ACES, including group times and content, how the Recovery Goals are used in DBT-ACES individual therapy, the Career Activities and Work as Therapy contingencies, and the DBT-ACES Diary Card. The interviewer should also prepare the client for the fact that the work contingencies and individual therapy will create intense pressure and require exposure experiences and willingness that they need to be sure they want to take on.

Pretreatment Step 6: The Decision to Proceed to DBT-ACES

Based on the successful completion of the DBT-ACES pretreatment process, the client is either accepted or given the task to resolve the DBT-ACES-interfering behavior(s). If accepted, they are told that the team approves the client into DBT-ACES and asked if and when they would like to attend. This is not a trivial decision. Often it is strategic not to let the client decide right in that moment, and instead to take time to consider further and discuss with others in their life whose opinion they respect. Again, there is a big difference between SDBT and DBT-ACES, and clients who see DBT-ACES as the only path to keeping their therapist may agree even though it isn't their Wise Mind. In such cases, the interviewer may be the one with the outside perspective to help the therapist and client negotiate this situation.

It is also important to help the client decide when to start DBT-ACES. As previously mentioned, at the beginning of SDBT, the client likely felt awful and desperate, and their life was likely chaotic and unstable. Generally, to meet DBT-ACES criteria, this has dramatically changed, and they are feeling better than they have in a long time. Thus, they may want to consider taking a break and relaxing into the gains they have made, rather than jumping into a high-pressure program for another year. On the other hand, many clients have momentum now and want to keep it and/or their relationship with their individual therapist going. It is also possible that the client could have future plans that would take them out of the area or otherwise make it hard to participate later. In any case, pushing the client (and their individual SDBT therapist) to make this decision explicitly rather than just implicitly is key. We absolutely want them—and ideally right away—yet making this harder to achieve leads to a stronger commitment and better outcome. And, generally, clients only complete the DBT-ACES program once. So, if the client is not ready or now is not good timing, we recommend that they wait.

Either during the application and DBT-ACES interview or in a subsequent interview, the client who is about to start DBT-ACES should meet with a DBT-ACES group leader to be sure the client is clear on the skills curriculum, format, and expectations. Again, the focus is on orienting, troubleshooting, and increasing commitment.

Overall, the DBT-ACES pretreatment process is fairly lengthy, and it is worth acknowledging for the client how daunting the process might seem. It is important to accept that this will be too much for some clients. Given the client's life circumstances, a comprehensive DBT-ACES program or working at a living wage and getting off of disability might not be the right fit for them. Thus, the process of DBT-ACES pretreatment should be characterized by validation as well as highlighting dialectical tensions and working toward synthesis and Wise Mind.

If the client has participated in SDBT at another DBT program (not the one where DBT-ACES is being offered) or at some time in the past, it is still recommended they complete as much of the DBT-ACES pretreatment process as they can. The limiting factor usually is the performance evaluations from their group and individual therapists, but this can usually be resolved at intake for the DBT-ACES program. For example, clients who have recently completed SDBT in an outside program and are applying to DBT-ACES can be asked to contact their previous SDBT individual and group therapists to complete the performance evaluations. If the client is currently in an outside SDBT program and is therefore completing the DBT-ACES pretreatment with their SDBT therapist as well as the DBT-ACES intake contact, the key is ensuring that the SDBT therapist understands what is involved in DBT-ACES and the pretreatment process so they can participate effectively. Intake staff can do the DBT-ACES interview or delegate that to another DBT clinician or the DBT-ACES group leader.

In summary, because the comprehensive DBT-ACES program is designed for individuals with long-standing unemployment or underemployment issues who are disabled by their emotional and/or psychiatric problems and has multiple requirements that clients will find challenging, we have developed these pretreatment steps to be sure they are ready to take this on. One or more pretreatment steps can also be used as needed in a DBT program that wants to implement DBT Next Steps strategies depending on what seems valuable for that DBT program or on a case-by-case basis. When to implement DBT-ACES as a comprehensive program versus some or all of DBT Next Steps is considered more broadly in the next chapter.

CHAPTER 13

DBT Next Steps or DBT-ACES

Incorporating the Model in Full or in Parts

This chapter considers how a DBT therapist or program can incorporate DBT Next Steps. Three options are reviewed: (1) incorporating one or more DBT Next Steps strategies as make sense within an SDBT program; (2) incorporating DBT Next Steps as a package as clients move down the hierarchy and the focus is on avoidance of behaviors needed to achieve their goals; and (3) implementing a DBT-ACES comprehensive program.

Incorporating DBT Next Steps Strategies into DBT

There are many advantages to integrating only certain DBT Next Steps strategies to complement a cognitive-behavioral treatment plan, an SDBT program, or a DBT graduate group. For one, doing so allows for ultimate flexibility, as well as offering a lower-dose option. This is desirable for many SDBT graduates and is applicable for clients who are largely thriving and already pursuing many of the Recovery Goals that are a part of DBT Next Steps. The intensity of a two-session per week treatment program might not be necessary for clients based on the severity of their avoidance behaviors, or perhaps more importantly, how many life worth living goals they have already achieved.

Many of the strategies listed in this book can be used to increase employment and overall self-sufficiency among clients without a comprehensive DBT-ACES program, particularly in standard care settings that offer a range of cognitive-behavioral therapies including SDBT (Carmel & Comtois, 2023). Examples of strategies and skills that work on their own include the Recovery Goals; the work contingencies (Normative Productivity, Work as Therapy, or Career Activities); the DBT Next Steps skills (individually, as modules, or as a complete curriculum); and the DBT Next Steps Check-In.

One limitation of adapting Next Steps without the comprehensive model is that the strategies work in tandem. For instance, the work contingencies are an active ingredient in DBT Next Steps—structured activities that move the client toward financial independence, building gradually within a clear time frame. Removing these contingencies weakens motivation for clients to demonstrate new behaviors. A program that uses the Check-In practice and teaches the DBT Next Steps Skills-Training curriculum while not maintaining these contingencies runs the risk of clients not having sufficient motivation to use the skills to make meaningful changes. Remember, "Contingencies create capabilities."

Programs that are considering implementing DBT Next Steps in any capacity might consider a synthesis of integrating only certain strategies while tracking clinical outcomes and acceptability among clinical staff. This will provide the data needed to guide decisions to expand to other strategies or skills. Normative Productivity hours are a natural starting point for the SDBT program that wants to adopt DBT Next Steps and is uncertain about where to start or finds the multiple strategies daunting. Normative Productivity requirements are not that different from what most DBT therapists are encouraging their clients to do. It's an added time frame and consequences for not accumulating structured, scheduled social activities. When Normative Productivity requirements are folded into an SDBT program, it turbocharges the client's move toward a more behaviorally activated life that then enables them to go out and pursue a range of life worth living goals not limited to work or school. It is also acceptable for therapists, as it doesn't set the bar high while still functioning as a contingency for the therapist who doesn't want to lose their client to a therapy suspension (once again, contingencies create capabilities—this time, for the therapist). In our experience, clients have more success with DBT Next Steps when they approach it with Normative Productivity hours already built in. Similarly, programs have more success with DBT Next Steps when they integrate Normative Productivity as one of the first components, evaluate the therapeutic benefit and staff acceptability, and then build on it. Remember our metaphor: It's easier to climb the mountain if you have hiking shoes broken in and that have already scaled a few foothills first.

Another strategy that works well alone is the Recovery Goals (Chapter 4) since they offer an effective way to organize targets for many clients who want to increase self-sufficiency or pursue school or employment goals. Getting a job, finding friends, or getting a degree are often DBT targets that are too vague and multilayered to be effective. The therapist and client take stabs at such a big target from different directions, but the dyad often struggles to make meaningful headway and gets discouraged. The Recovery Goals self-assessment exercise helps the therapist and client to unpack what is involved in employment and self-sufficiency and decide what are already strengths for the client, what is partially in place, and where there might be a long way to go. This behavioral specificity provides a structure to get DBT moving again. The Recovery Goals can be paired with the use of *in vivo* exposure that is critical in helping clients move into new territory and take chances, such as applying for work, moving into their own home, or finding friends or a relationship. *In vivo* exposure to new adventures stands in contrast to other exposure-based adaptations of DBT with which DBT therapists are familiar but that focus more on exposure to past events.

The DBT Next Steps skills modules can be integrated into individual or group sessions to target problem behaviors and address particular skills deficits, such as increasing tools for effective time management and reducing perfectionism that can be immobilizing for many clients. Programs can select skills modules from the curriculum to fit the needs of a clinical population, such as adding Alternatives to Perfectionism skills (Chapter 15) in a DBT for Eating Disorders program targeting rigid standards of oneself and critical evaluations of one's performance. Community Mapping from the Establishing and Re-Evaluating Relationships module (Chapter 16) can be added to a DBT–Substance Use Disorder program that is tasked with helping clients in recovery to build new bridges, create community reinforcement, and embed themselves in new social settings where drug use isn't the focus. Many skills modules are well-suited to a DBT graduate group model that expands on SDBT skills and keeps them from getting rusty. This includes the Managing Emotions Effectively and Applications of Mindfulness modules (Chapters 18 and 20) that focus on strengthening and generalizing SDBT skills modules in a range of new environments. For example, the Assessment of Reducing Vulnerability Skills: What's Working and What's Not and How to Change It from the Managing Emotions Effectively module works to assess, problem-solve, and troubleshoot the process of integrating emotion regulation skills into a client's day-to-day life. The Applications of Mindfulness module features skills to build in structured and scheduled mindfulness practice to increase centeredness, decrease emotional reactivity, and proactively target rumination.

Another strategy to consider on its own is the group-based component of the DBT Next Steps Check-In (Chapter 14). This process offers a natural focus on Action Steps toward values and quality-of-life (QOL) goals that is well suited to a DBT graduate group program, individual therapy with a client who is not making progress, or other skills-based groups outside of DBT. The Check-In process teaches clients to be effective problem-solvers by repeatedly and collaboratively setting achievable Action Steps in the service of long-term goals, blocking avoidance, and reinforcing action. In the group context, all the group members are viewing the process objectively when they observe and help each other, as well as subjectively by doing their own Check-In. With group leaders joining in the process as well, the environment offers opportunities to model effective means of setting Action Steps and for troubleshooting. Outside of a group setting, Check-In can also be incorporated into SDBT individual therapy to more clearly and precisely target QOL skills and avoidance while reinforcing progress.

Moving from SDBT to DBT Next Steps Informally

A program might see the value in DBT Next Steps for patients who have moved from reducing out-of-control behaviors to targeting avoidance and increasing certain positive behaviors. The DBT Next Steps strategies might be implemented for clients as they reach this stage of treatment. In such a circumstance, individual therapist–client dyads gradually pick up Next Steps approaches and a DBT Next Steps group can be available for clients, but it is not treated as a separate program requiring an explicit decision to enter through a formal pretreatment process and doesn't have an explicit time limit or other formal structure. In this way, it is incorporated like other evidence-based modalities in DBT—a client has a problem with *X* so the treatment for *X* is incorporated into SDBT.

While the informal incorporation of DBT Next Steps into SDBT has not been evaluated as DBT-ACES has, there are a few situations where it might be the best path. The first is a smaller DBT program where there are not enough clients needing DBT Next Steps at the same time to set up or maintain a comprehensive DBT-ACES program. In other cases, this approach might be exciting to some DBT team members and not others, and it is easier and more practical for therapists who are motivated to use DBT Next Steps to do so. Finally, some DBT programs of independent practitioners organize their practices differently, like seeing patients over long periods, seeing younger patients, or focusing on specific issues, such as eating disorders. While the program may be large, it is also very diverse and there may not be enough patients to maintain a distinct program continuously.

Adopting the Comprehensive DBT-ACES Model

Of course, the alternative is to adopt DBT-ACES and implement the comprehensive model. The SDBT program that chooses to stretch its limits to incorporate comprehensive DBT-ACES will likely experience a similar pattern of growth and development that it went through while implementing SDBT. Essentially, one needs to get SDBT teams on board with DBT-ACES as one did to launch SDBT in the first place.

Comtois, Koons, et al. (2007) note:

> Swimming against the current, while necessary to apply DBT, is both challenging and wearing for the therapist. This is particularly true early in the implementation process before there is clinic-specific evidence that DBT works at the local level. It can be still harder in public-sector systems serving psychiatrically disabled clients accustomed to receiving services "from cradle to grave." Given that DBT represents a paradigm shift for many, it can help to orient people (e.g., staff, administrators, clients, spouses, and parents) ahead of time to the message that doing DBT may mean doing things radically differently from the ways to which they are accustomed. Before embarking on building a DBT program (and certainly as new staff and clients join the program), we suggest getting an individual commitment from all of these individuals to doing DBT. (p. 39)

As in SDBT, engaging administration and clinic management with orienting and commitment is key to a successful launch of DBT-ACES. This often involves sharing the published effectiveness and cost–benefit analysis research to justify the continuation of an intensive program. It is notable that evaluations of DBT-ACES have demonstrated outcomes comparable to those of clinical trials, with promising findings for increasing school and work activities and substantial cost benefits. The results of the initial feasibility trial found that clients in DBT–ACES were three times more likely to be working or in school and five times more likely to be working 20 hours a week or more in the year of DBT-ACES than their SDBT year (Comtois et al., 2010). A three-site evaluation replicated and exceeded these pre–post results and included a cost–benefit analysis yielding substantial savings of over $17,000 per DBT-ACES client compared to the year prior to SDBT, with cost offset primarily driven by the decrease in inpatient utilization but also an independent monetary benefit from client work and school productivity (Carmel et al., 2021; Comtois et al., 2020).

An SDBT program interested in adopting DBT-ACES is encouraged to provide SDBT for a fixed duration of time and to integrate the Normative Productivity contingency within SDBT. This sets clients up for success when they enter into DBT-ACES. Our program at the University of Washington offers 12 months of SDBT, with a discussion between individual therapist and client at the 6-month mark (informally called a "state-of-the-union" on our team) to ensure that there is sufficient therapeutic progress to continue in SDBT for the full 12 months. Orienting to

DBT-ACES happens around this discussion at the 6-month mark of SDBT so that the client has sufficient time to understand the expectations and consider whether it's in their Wise Mind to apply to DBT-ACES. Once a client graduates after 12 months of SDBT in our program, they are unable to return to SDBT. The only option for additional DBT services in the clinic is to apply to DBT-ACES (which is an open-ended option--a patient could return for DBT-ACES years after their graduation from SDBT).

Part of commitment to adopt DBT-ACES entails problem solving for the clients who do not complete DBT-ACES. Proper use of contingencies in DBT Next Steps does require support from the larger clinic to discharge or refer clients who drop out of treatment or go on suspension, in a similar way that SDBT programs must have a plan for discharging or referring clients who drop out of SDBT due to the four-miss rule. With the increased expectations of DBT-ACES, it's worth noting that clients can drop out of DBT-ACES for a lot more factors, including not returning after suspension for failure to meet the requirements of Normative Productivity, Work as Therapy, or Career Activities (see Table 11.2). A resurgence of life-threatening behavior leads to an ongoing probation status. A DBT-ACES program will need to figure out discharge or referral options for the clients who move from suspension or probation to dropping out, as well as creating a path for them to return to DBT-ACES to resume therapy. For the client who reapplies, we recommend an extended pretreatment phase to problem-solve and troubleshoot what led to their previously dropping out, such that the client now stands a better chance of succeeding in the program after the issues that interfered previously have been resolved. For example, one client who dropped out due to nonattendance and lateness was asked to demonstrate her ability to reengage in DBT-ACES by stopping by the clinic at a set time for 4 consecutive weeks in a row. Once she demonstrated the ability to show up on time consistently by making an appearance in the clinic lobby for a few minutes, the consultation team proceeded with accepting her application to return to DBT-ACES.

When a program has a policy that clients who graduate from SDBT are unable to reenter SDBT again in the future, this reduces the chance that dysfunctional client behaviors get reinforced. For the client who has dropped out of DBT-ACES following re-occurrences of suicidal behavior, their return to SDBT would shift the treatment to remove behavioral expectations such Work as Therapy. This withdrawal of expectations would occur following the suicidal behavior, thus resulting in its negative reinforcement. Resuming SDBT would likely be extending the duration of treatment, which can be a strong reinforcer for many clients. Remember, "Contingencies create capabilities." Programs aren't making it easier for the client to succeed by being more nurturing or flexible in response to a re-occurrence of escalated behavior, or by withdrawing behavioral expectations in the face of it.

Given these numerous factors for orienting, commitment, and problem-solving implementation barriers, it's also important to highlight the fact that DBT-ACES is fundamentally DBT. Even with the changes noted above, there is no change to the structure of the program; therefore, implementing DBT-ACES is not radically different than establishing an SDBT program. All of the four modes of SDBT treatment remain the same (albeit with different QOL targets focused on the Recovery Goals, rather than life-threatening behaviors). Successful orienting requires reminders of this: When it comes down to it, there are not many changes required for the SDBT program looking to adopt DBT-ACES.

A primary dialectical stance is to implement the DBT-ACES comprehensive model while simultaneously considering ways to modify it in order to best meet the needs and limitations of both the setting and clinical population. This involves a responsiveness to the initial program evaluations of DBT-ACES and examining client outcomes and acceptability among clients and staff. Teams can consider functional validation of ideas that emerge for modifying DBT-ACES to best support clients as they cross the divide between wanting financial independence and making it happen.

Whatever turns out to be the best approach to integrating DBT Next Steps into a DBT therapist or program's repertoire, it is hoped that the DBT Next Steps strategies (i.e., Part II of this book) will benefit DBT therapists targeting QOL-interfering behaviors that have gotten into murky territory—often because they require an increase in behavior and blocking avoidance. Ironically, as challenging as life-threatening behaviors, nonattendance and noncompliance TIBs, and high-risk QOL-interfering behaviors are to the general therapist, they are often relatively easy for DBT therapists and the bread and butter of the work. Mobilizing a client who is stable but stuck, however, requires a greater emphasis on *in vivo* exposure, contingency management approaches, and didactic strategies that are not typically the focus of SDBT. We hope the reader has found more clarity, precision, and compassion for how to do this.

The final part of this book moves from DBT Next Steps strategies for the therapist to DBT Next Step skills. Part IV provides detailed lesson plans for teaching DBT Next Step skills-training groups that correspond to our companion volume, *DBT Next Steps Skills Handouts.*

PART IV

THE DBT-ACES SKILLS CURRICULUM

CHAPTER 14

Overview of DBT Next Steps Skills Format and Strategies

In Part II of this book, we reviewed all of the DBT Next Steps principles and strategies. Thus, in Part IV, we focus on "what to do and how to do it" rather than underlying principles. If you are trying to figure out why a skill or a skills group procedure is set up as it is, please refer back to the principles in Part II, particularly Chapter 5, on skills training, or you can review the case studies in Chapter 3 to see how these strategies apply clinically.

Core Principles

1. The primary goal of the DBT Next Steps Skills Curriculum is for clients to learn to be their own therapist (at least as it relates to general mental health stability). Specific capabilities include being able to:
   - Mix and match skills—that is, to assess a problem and match skills to it, not just see a skill and match problems to it (as in SDBT skills training).
   - Understand explicitly what they experience implicitly in individual therapy, including behavioral assessment, reinforcement, goal setting, problem solving, troubleshooting, cognitive restructuring, and dialectics, and be able to apply it on themself and their environment.
   - Understand explicitly the steps needed to create their own social support system and effectively interact with people at work, new and established friends, and treatment providers.
   - Develop proficiency in these skills through repeated practice.

2. Similar to the difference between undergraduate and graduate training, in undergraduate school you learn subject matter in theory and in graduate school you learn to apply what you have learned in structured practice and to become a practitioner yourself with the ability to teach others. In DBT Next Steps, the Career Activities, Work as Therapy, and Check-In for DBT Next Steps are like practica and internships in graduate school.
3. DBT Next Steps uses a skills-training curriculum linked to Recovery Goals (see Chapter 4). The DBT Next Steps skills-training modules and handouts described in this manual teach:
   - More applied versions of the SDBT skills
   - Other CBT skills such as goal setting, problem solving, and contingency management
   - Specific interpersonal skills to use to function effectively at work, with health care providers, and to establish oneself in a supportive community outside of mental health
   - Strategies to overcome typical problems of individuals on psychiatric disability, including rigid or perfectionistic thinking, time mismanagement, anxiety, anger, and depression
   - Balance of acceptance-based skills modules (e.g., Applications of Mindfulness) with change-based skills modules (e.g., Managing Emotions Effectively)
4. Clients are expected to behave in DBT Next Steps skills training as if attending a college course or at a training for work with their supervisor present. They should dress appropriately for their career plans. The group leaders coach clients with regard to this expectation, set contingencies, and reinforce effective behavior.

Format of the Skills-Training Modules

1. Modules are 1 month long, based on a 4-week month. As certain months have 5 weeks, the group leaders decide what material is worth expanding on and do more on that or teach something related to material from another source. For a fifth week, make up new assignments, repeat an assignment, or give an assignment vacation.
2. There are six skills modules, which can be offered once or twice. We have generally offered them twice so that, as in SDBT, clients go through the skills curriculum twice in 1 year. The order of modules is not fixed, but this order has been effective for us in our Harborview program:
   - Perfectionism versus Reinforcement
   - Establishing and Re-Evaluating Relationships
   - Time Management
   - Managing Emotions Effectively
   - Succeeding after DBT
   - Applications of Mindfulness
3. There are client handouts and teaching points for each module. In the sections that follow, the teaching points for each module are described week by week and refer to the client materials in the companion volume, *DBT Next Steps Skills Handouts*. Note in the companion volume that there is a blank for the months each module will be taught, and the skills

leaders should ask the clients to put in the months that match for when they will be learning each module.

4. Client handouts for each module start with a syllabus sheet that lists the topics for each week and the assignment associated with each teaching topic. Participants are, therefore, preinformed of the assignments and expected to independently keep up with the material even if they miss a week (just as in college or at work).

Assignments

1. In DBT Next Steps, the word "assignments" is used instead of "homework" or "worksheets" because this word is more general to work, not just school contexts.
2. Assignments in DBT Next Steps should always be completed in writing ahead of time, as this is the expectation of most job and school programs and leads to more thorough understanding of the material. Also, writing notes during class and during review of assignments provides the client with a completed notebook and relevant correct examples at the end of the year. Thus, the *DBT Next Steps Skills Handouts* volume will serve as a reference in the future.
3. Assignments are expected to be completed for each week, even if the client missed the class or the assignment was done but not written down for a previous class. Our goal is to introduce a range of skills that may be helpful now, and to which the client can return in the months and years after graduation when a problem in that area arises. Complete, written assignments that are corrected as needed during assignment review ensure that the clients (a) practice each skill that we teach so they are sure they understand them and are able to ask questions and get corrections, (b) know what the pros and cons of that skill are, and (c) have correct notes in their skills book for reference after graduation.
4. If assignments are not done, they should be completed in writing and turned into the skills co-leader as soon as possible. If the client did the assignment and did not write it down, the client can report this during group and is still asked to write it out for review by the skills co-leader at the next group.
5. Clients are oriented to the need for complete, written assignments as they are oriented to DBT Next Steps. Clients are also oriented to treat these assignments as they would at work or in college: Do assignments completely, on time, neatly, and be ready to discuss them. If they do not complete assignments on time, clients are oriented that, as in a work or college situation, they need to take the initiative to catch the skills co-leader at an appropriate time (e.g., at a break, before class) to show them that the assignments are complete and ask any questions about their assignments. (This role is for the skills co-leader, not the skills leader in charge of the primary teaching.) The skills co-leader is not expected to have to chase down clients to get their assignments.
6. At the same time, the skills co-leader should maintain at least a general track record of how many assignments the clients are behind. If they are four or more behind, they are suspended from DBT Next Steps skills class until they are caught up. We recommend that clients sit in the lobby and complete assignments until they are caught up and then join

group as soon as they are fewer than four assignments behind. As discussed in Chapter 5, the skills co-leader needs to be both on top of whether clients are behind and avoid becoming burned out by tracking assignments.

7. If clients have questions about getting themselves to do the assignment or have complaints about the assignment, they should take these to the individual therapist who functions as a private coach to the client—just as we would not want the client to bring complaints or statements of general inability to their boss or professor during a meeting or class. They should primarily practice GIVE and DEAR MAN skills with their skills leaders.
8. In class, review assignments for correctness, completeness, and mindfulness. It is also a continuation of the teaching and an opportunity to fine-tune clients' understanding and increase their troubleshooting with this skill. In reviewing assignments, it is important to reinforce effective assignments and, in particular, ambitious or thorough assignments and creativity. Generally, this is done with validation, praise, irreverence, or another light strategy that is an effective reinforcer for that client. (One goal of DBT Next Steps is to learn how to "read a room" and be able to see what reinforces others and use reinforcers flexibly with different people. Now is a good chance for skills leaders to model this skill.)
9. Several assignments throughout the year involve the clients interviewing or role-playing situations with their individual therapist. Be sure that the individual therapists in DBT Next Steps are oriented and committed to doing such assignments before they are assigned. It is also helpful if the skills leaders remind individual therapists when such assignments are upcoming so individual therapists can pace the sessions accordingly.
10. It is helpful if skills leaders have a system of communicating with individual therapists about attendance, assignment completion, and the behavioral effectiveness of their clients so they can help clients be successful in group. We alternately use our secure email system or make a worksheet that we copy and put in therapists' mailboxes after group (a template for the group email is available in Appendix A: Sample Completed DBT Next Steps Skills-Training Class Notes). Alternatively, DBT Next Steps individual therapists can gather this information in individual sessions when checking on other therapy modes.

Practice Professional Behavior in DBT Next Steps and DBT-ACES Next Steps Requirements toward the Recovery Goals Handouts

1. As part of the DBT Next Steps Interview, the Practice Professional Behavior in DBT Next Steps and DBT-ACES Requirements toward the Recovery Goals handouts, as well as all the other "DBT Next Steps Overview" materials in the *DBT Next Steps Skills Handouts* volume, should be reviewed. Therefore, it is not necessary to take group time to review these handouts.
2. Should there be confusion or an increase in unprofessional behavior in the group, the skills group leaders should re-orient the skills group to these expectations. If only one or two people are engaging in unprofessional behavior, this can happen at break or via a phone call during the week.

Introduction and Graduation

Introduction of New Clients

1. New clients enter DBT Next Steps only on the first class of the month (e.g., our DBT Next Steps class is Thursday at 3 P.M., so new clients enter only on the first Thursday of the month).
2. The DBT Next Steps syllabus (see the "DBT Next Steps Overview" in *DBT Next Steps Skills Handouts*) lists the group format and tentative timing as well as the schedule of modules. The DBT Next Steps Skills Group Participation Guidelines provide orientation and coaching hints to clients about how to participate in each section of skills-training class.
3. When new clients join, we start with everyone introducing themselves. Skills leaders not known to the client can introduce themselves first. Client introductions go in the order of seniority, beginning with members who have been in class the longest. Each client is prompted to state:
   - Their name (and pronouns, if desired)
   - How long they have been in DBT Next Steps
   - What brought them to SDBT in the first place (using generalities rather than talking about suicidal behavior, but DBT Next Steps clients know the drill, so this doesn't need to be said, just stopped if needed)
   - What has changed for the better since they have been in SDBT and DBT Next Steps
   - Where they are going/what DBT Next Steps is doing to help them get there

   If clients fail to mention an obvious achievement like a job, award, or enrolling in a school program, the skills leaders can prompt for this information. Self-invalidation should be overtly blocked without spending time discussing it.
4. As the skills leader moves through the stages of new members' first group, details about how each stage works should be noted with reference to the DBT Next Steps Skills Group Participation Guidelines—for instance:

   > "First we do Good News. This means finding something in our life that went well, something we are grateful for, something exciting going on. If your mind goes blank because in this moment things seem dark and you can't think of Good News—just tell us about what is not wrong. We'll all go first so you can get the sense of it. [Everyone shares their Good News.] So, get the idea? What is your Good News this week?"

   The same process applies for Check-In, although we allow clients to take 1–3 weeks of just listening to others check in to get in the loop. They don't usually wait that long to participate, but it helps to take the pressure off. We also recommend they work with their individual therapist on their first ambition and Action Steps for Check-In. Orient new clients to just listen during assignment review; otherwise, new clients who feel unjustified guilt, shame, or anxiety about not having completed the assignment may try and jump in, which is not very effective for anyone. For new material, orient to the syllabus, which is the front page of each module and lists all the assignments due that month.
5. Remind clients that all assignments are written and due whether or not you were in group

the previous week. Also be sure they understand that they can't be four or more assignments behind and discuss how to submit back assignments to the skills co-leader (as discussed in Assignments above as well as in Chapter 5). Orienting to this during the introduction of new clients is important, to ensure everyone is clear and there are no surprises if a group member is asked to leave to catch up on their assignments.

Graduation from DBT Next Steps Skills-Training Group

1. Completion of either 6 months or a year of DBT Next Steps constitutes criteria for graduation. This can be decided as a program, with the duration more flexible depending on the clients. For example, our Harborview program is 1 year with two trips through the DBT Next Steps Skills Curriculum, but a program for teens who are used to learning and need to move on to college might be 6 months, with only one time through the skills. Duration should be decided at pretreatment, not on the fly.
2. The graduation of each client should be celebrated.
   - The goal of graduation is to observe and describe success and future plans, and is important reinforcement not only for the graduating client but also for any family or guests they invite to attend, other DBT Next Steps clients, and the DBT team.
   - Graduations should be anticipated at least 2 months in advance to be sure the clients are prepared. They are also asked what refreshments they would most like for their graduation (not a requirement, but a Harborview DBT-ACES tradition). If the budget allows, these can be provided; otherwise, group members can bring a potluck meal.
   - Clients and their individual therapists can decide if they want the DBT Next Steps group graduation to be their last DBT Next Steps session, or whether they would like to continue with their individual therapist for 1–3 more weeks. The preferences of clients and therapists vary, so there is no wrong choice here.
   - Graduations are generally celebrated in the last half-hour of DBT Next Steps group following the break (longer if more than one person is graduating that day). The first half of group covers the new material, but the Check-In is skipped for that week. Clients are reminded they should do their own Check-In and pick their own target to work on for the next week.
   - Clients and invited family or friends are oriented to bring a concrete expression of congratulations or a goodbye card or present, although they don't have to. This is a case for Wise Mind regarding their preference and their relationship with the graduating client. Staff may also give their own cards or gifts if that reflects their relationship with the client (in accordance with SDBT manual principles on gifts as well as agency guidelines).
3. The typical graduation format is as follows:
   a. All DBT team members, DBT Next Steps clients, and anyone else the client would like to invite to their graduation.
   b. Food is provided, and some portion of the event presents an informal opportunity for the graduating client to say goodbye and for the team to highlight what they have achieved during the year.

c. A more formal section should include an opportunity to:
   i. Give the client a certificate of graduation signed by the group leaders, individual therapist, and/or clinic director or prescriber.
   ii. Allow the client to say what they would like to express.
   iii. Allow the DBT staff to highlight the client's achievements and say goodbye.
   iv. Allow the other clients and guests to make any comments they would like.

Flow of the DBT Next Steps Skills Group Session

As described in Chapter 5, "Skills Training," each 2-hour session of DBT Next Steps skills starts with Good News and then moves to the Check-In practice, Review of Assignments, and then Review of New Material. A break is taken about half-way at a natural point to pause. Before, after, or at break, clients with incomplete assignments can review them with the co-leader. Chapter 5 presented skills training in general, with a focus on why things are done as they are. The following section provides pragmatic details of how to implement a DBT Next Steps group session that should be considered in the context of the principles discussed in Chapter 5.

Starting the DBT Next Steps Group Sessions

1. It is important to set the right tone for the start of group to mirror what would be expected at the beginning of a seminar class or staff meeting—lots of GIVE, particularly Easy Manner. If clients present in ways that would be likely to lead to negative consequences in the work or school setting they aspire to (e.g., visibly depressed or anxious body language, sharing too much information, avoiding eye contact or small talk by looking only at their phone), the group leaders should prompt for more effective interpersonal behavior.
2. It is important to be sensitive to the setting in which the client aspires to be. What is expected in a staff meeting at a law office, a construction site, busy cardiac unit in a hospital, high school, military base, day care center, and big box store will be quite different. Expectations for classes during freshman year at a community college, a vocational culinary arts program, a physical therapy program at a state university, trucking school, and an arts program at a private college are equally different. Co-leaders also need to be sensitive to the culture of the client and their workplace as interpersonal norms differ a lot. This is where a dialectical philosophy, radical acceptance, and mindfulness WHAT and HOW skills as well as GIVE skills are needed by co-leaders and clients. Modeling and coaching of clients to "read the room" and be open to who other clients are and where they intend to work or go to school can be important. In summary, we accept that there are limits to what any set of co-leaders and clients can do on the one hand, and we strive for clients to be skillful with many different people, norms, and circumstances and to practice this in the group where they can receive feedback.
3. To promote this positive attitude, instead of traditional mindfulness, DBT Next Steps groups lead with Good News. Everyone, clients and co-leaders included, prepares some Good News to share with the group at the beginning of the session. Someone volunteers

(or is volunteered) to start, and we go around the physical room or "popcorn" around the virtual room if group is happening through telehealth. Clients report on what has gone well for them that week, something challenging they achieved, a windfall, something they are grateful for—the point is that the discussion is positive.

4. If clients include negative as well as positive news in their Good News or include self-validation, the leaders should use an Easy Manner to restate the Good News with the positive alone or ask the client to do so. For instance, if the client said, "Not really a big deal, but my manager gave me a high five for getting my work done early," the leader could say, "A high five! That's great!" or "Whoops—bit of self-invalidation slipped in there . . . say that again without the 'not really a big deal' part," and offer "That's great!" to the Good News alone.
5. If a client can't think of any Good News, they are asked to say something that is not wrong instead of passing. For instance, they could say, "The bus was on time" or "The sun is out" or "My shoes don't pinch." With the repeated expectation of Good News, clients are shaped to notice what is going well, what is not wrong, and are more likely to share that with others.

DBT Next Steps Check-In Practice

1. Goals of the Check-In (which can be highlighted to clients periodically):
    a. The Check-In practice is designed to help a client identify a long-term ambition that they are actually committed to achieving, learn how to identify Action Steps that are feasible yet challenging to work toward the ambition, and learn which ones are effective and avoidant behaviors that facilitate or get in the way of achieving Action Steps.
    b. Check-In encourages the core principle of "learning to be your own therapist" and learning self-sufficiency.
    c. Check-In treats many other problems, including perfectionism, hopelessness, helplessness, willfulness, self-invalidation, and self-punishment in response to mistakes.
    d. Directly targeting phobic avoidance of grand ambitions teaches clients to allow for possibilities.
    e. Check-In teaches clients to nonjudgmentally and openly self-observe their own effective and problematic behaviors so they can identify potential problems early—often before they even occur.
    f. It teaches clients to effectively and quickly generate alternatives and to recognize small improvements so they do not jump ship before they can succeed.
    g. Check-In focuses on building on success: choosing Action Steps that are the next logical steps that are sufficiently challenging to feel some pride of accomplishment (and get reinforcement from the group), yet not so challenging that they violate the shaping law that breeds success.
2. General Principles and Structure:
    a. Each client and skills leader participates in Check-In each week. Generally, someone volunteers (or is volunteered) to start, and then the Check-In continues around the physical room or "popcorns," or goes alphabetically around the virtual telehealth room.

b. Skills leaders should use a "coping model" for their Check-In, referring to ambitions and Action Steps where they are not going to be perfectly successful ("mastery model") or likely to have serious problems ("failure model"). Skills leaders also follow the DBT principles for personal self-disclosure and observing therapist limits as part of their Check-In. Typical Check-In topics for therapists are exercise, diet, or other health behaviors, mindfulness, and organizational improvement. Therapists should not choose something likely to be particularly upsetting to clients, as this will distract them from the process.

c. There are two versions of the Check-In form: long and short (see the "DBT Next Steps Overview" in *DBT Next Steps Skills Handouts*). The long form includes details on each step of the Check-In and is recommended for new clients for at least the first couple of months (longer if they don't have the concepts clear). After that, the short form is often preferred by clients as it gives them more room to write and is less cluttered.

d. Check-In forms should be completed in writing before group starts by all clients unless/until they have the sheet and the steps sufficiently mastered that they can do the process by memory quickly, smoothly, and correctly. If they are still stumbling, tangential, vague, have steps incorrectly described, or are otherwise not prepared, they should be directed to go back to a written preparation before group.

e. If a client (or leader) wants to change their ambition or Action Step, they should *not* do so in the middle of a week. Everyone is responsible for the Action Steps they commit to for their Check-In. If they want to plan a change for the following week, they can discuss it at the "new Action Step" stage of the Check-In. Meanwhile, they should do their best to complete what they originally committed to the previous week.

f. New clients to DBT Next Steps are not expected to participate in the Check-In for the first or second week. Instead, they are expected to nonjudgmentally observe what others have done and discuss options with their individual therapist. Their first presentation of their ambitions and Action Steps should just establish what they are. When they have done that, they can start working on them and reporting with the rest of the group.

3. Elements of the Check-In:

a. There are multiple elements to a check-in that are described in detail. While a lot of explanation occurs here to ensure that leaders understand what skills are involved, in reality, the Check-Ins go fairly quickly unless someone is struggling with doing their Action Steps as long as clients prepare for their Check-In ahead of time.

b. *Ambition:* An ambition is not something to achieve now. It is what the client is passionate about achieving as a substantial and permanent change in their life. *DBT Next Steps Skills Handouts* includes a sample ambition in Appendix 3 for reference.

i. An ambition is not the means to an end, but an end in itself.

ii. An ambition could be accomplished in a couple of months, a couple of years, or a decade. The commitment to the ambition is more important than the time frame.

iii. *Example ambitions:* Being a radiology technician, getting off disability, "traveling to see the solar eclipse in South Africa in 2030 with my boyfriend," getting married, financial independence, learning conversational Spanish in the next 2 years, buying a house, time with children who are in a partner's custody, a job, graduate school, lose

10% of my body weight, "want to be a competent artist/teacher who works for social change," "wake up respecting myself each morning," travel to the Eastern seaboard, learn a language, and so on.

iv. The ambition should be stated as specifically as possible, but not so specifically that it loses its meaning/passion. For example, for some clients, particularly those who are perfectionistic, the ambition of "feeling confident" would be too general and unclear when it was achieved. The ambition could be made more specific in several different ways: "believe I will not lose my job," "be so good at my job that I get promotions or job offers," "believe the majority of people in my life I respect like me too," "be asked on dates," and so forth. For other clients, feeling confident is the key and something more specific could detract from that goal, so further specificity is not needed.

v. There is an art to picking a strong ambition with a client. The client needs to have an affective response (e.g., excitement, peace, hope) to an ambition that reflects real and meaningful change in their lives.

vi. Many clinicians are cautious about encouraging ambitions they fear are too out of reach for the client. This teaches the clients that they are limited. Most clinicians are not good judges of what clients can do. In addition, clients are generally acutely responsive to the expectations of their environment and, if you expect them to achieve ambitious goals, it is more likely they will do so. If it becomes clear that an ambition is infeasible, the client will observe this for themself and can work with the individual therapist to accept and respond to the disappointment, grief, or frustration. Skills leaders who have doubts about their client's ability to achieve their ambitions should bring the issue to their consultation team and discuss. Especially if the skills leader has never used systematic behavioral strategies to change their own behavior, it can be helpful for the consultation team to work with the therapist to use the Check-In to choose an ambition the skills leader has not achieved before using the standards listed above (or all the therapists on the team might try the Check-In as a team). The consultation team can follow the Check-In process with the skills leader (or everyone) each week until a substantial part of their ambition is achieved so the skills leader (and other therapists) can see how effective this strategy is when applied consistently. (This might well be a different ambition than the skills leader would choose in group because personal disclosure of issues you are substantially struggling with is not great modeling. While picking something challenging and achieving it is the lesson we want the skills leader to learn in their consultation team, the skills leader might pick something easier to work on for the Check-In in skills group.)

c. *Action Steps* are a step or series of steps that the client will do between group meetings to progress with their ambition.

i. Action Steps should be stated in very specific terms. The group must agree that the Action Step is a next logical step and that there is a clear measurement of its completion. "Clean my apartment" is insufficiently specific unless the intent is for the entire apartment to be completely clean by the beginning of the next group. More specific Action Steps could include "clean the bathroom and kitchen," "spend 5 hours over the course of the week cleaning my apartment," or "clean to the point I would not be embarrassed to have guests." Similarly, "study for school" is too general. The more specific options are "I will study in a coffee shop twice this week for an hour each," "I will complete all my assignments on time," or "I will start on the final project and spend at least 2 hours on it." A useful question to ask is "How will you know when you are done?"

ii. Action Steps should be solely under the control of the client and not require follow-through from other people. For instance, the Action Step "go on a date with my partner" is partly based on the partner's behavior. Better Action Steps would be "invite my partner to go on a date," "plan out the date my partner agreed to," or "go on a date if my partner doesn't back out." Similar problems exist with such Action Steps as "schedule an appointment with my boss," "fix my account information at the bank," "borrow $50 from my mother," and so forth. These each need revisions so they are entirely under the client's control.

iii. Action Steps should follow the Chapter 7 guidelines on contingency management. We particularly rely on the reinforcement guidelines of Chapter 2, "Shaping," in the book *Don't Shoot the Dog* (Pryor, 2018), which we also recommend skills leaders read. Action Steps should be difficult, yet the client should have a 50% chance of pulling them off. Less than that means too small a chance for reinforcement and will lead to slower progress and higher risk of giving up. Higher than that might run the risk of self-invalidating when it isn't attainable. You can simply ask the client, "Is there a 50% chance you can do this?" or ask how often they have done what they said they would do in the past and establish a next step relative to their past behavior.

iv. If the client doesn't know what amount of the Action Step is a reasonable choice, an effective Action Step is to self-monitor the behavior for a week or two to establish a baseline. Self-monitoring may also have a positive impact in itself. An Action Step could, therefore, be "track on your Diary Card the number of minutes a day you spend cleaning your house" or "see how many times a week you walk." If the baseline is zero as the behavior is not in the person's repertoire, a first Action Step can be to go out and determine what they can do. They need to not try to do too much because they are establishing a baseline, not an extraordinary occurrence that would be infeasible to maintain or build on. For instance, "clean your house as much as you have time/energy to do this week" or "see how long you can comfortably ride the stationary bike at one time."

v. Setting an Action Step is an example of public commitment, which has its own power. A key aspect of this process is having the clients learn to commit to specific Action Steps, focus on them throughout the week, and achieve them reliably. As a group, they can learn how to reinforce effective and desirable behaviors in each other, so be sure that the entire group is aware of each other's Action Steps and that the client and skills co-leader write down the Action Steps. If the client returns having done a different or tangential version of their Action Step, the skills co-leader must reiterate what they agreed the Action Step would be last week and ask the client to report their progress on that. Other achievements can be reinforced, but the client needs to be directed to do the exact Action Step they agreed to take at the last group. If clients cannot reliably recall their Action Steps, problem-solving how to remember the specific details needs to be conducted at Check-In. If they're not improving with this coaching in group, the client should be directed to address this problem with their individual therapist. It should also be discussed in consultation team meetings, as being unclear or not tracking commitments may not only be a persistent TIB, but could also be a problem in the client's behavior at work or elsewhere.

d. *Action Steps versus Employment Steps*
   i. While the main focus of the Check-In is the Action Step, we have discovered that having an Employment Step, specifically for the Career Activities or Work as Therapy contingencies, can help the group focus on each other's Work as Therapy and Career Activities requirements, which the support from the skills group makes easier for the clients to achieve. The Check-In form includes both the Action Step and the Employment Step, but it is up to the skills leaders how much to address the Employment Step or leave this for individual therapy.
   ii. Clients should specify each week (or at least frequently) which Career Activities or Work as Therapy contingency deadline is coming up next and when. This keeps it in the client's and the group's mind.
   iii. If the client's Action Step is directly related to their next deadline for Career Activities or Work as Therapy, their Employment Step and Action Step are the same and don't require additional actions.
   iv. If the Action Step is not related to the Career Activities or Work as Therapy deadline, the client should specify their Employment Step as well. Due to limited time in group, it is expected that the Employment Step will be worked out with the individual therapist and only the Action Step will be worked out during group.

e. *Progress*
   i. Successes should always be reported and acknowledged before describing what was not accomplished, so clients ought to begin by reporting exactly what parts of their Action and Employment Steps from last week were completed.
   ii. This report of successes is the time for the skills leaders and clients to do/say reinforcing things as a response. (This is noted with an asterisk [*] on the Check-In form.) Some groups develop a culture of big responses, such as applause, while others have smaller reactions, such as smiles, "good job," or verbal validation. Any response that is reinforcing to the client should be encouraged by the skills leaders. If the reaction of the group does not appear to be reinforcing, this is an excellent opportunity for the skills leaders to teach about the importance of reinforcement matching the client ("reading the room") and encourage alternative reinforcement options for that client. On the other hand, exposure to praise can also be considered, and therapists can coach clients to practice the opposite action to unjustified embarrassment, self-consciousness, guilt, or shame. If the group is catatonic or otherwise not responsive to the person's achievements, they need to be rallied into creating an effective reinforcing response.

iii. Reinforcement is pointless if it is not observed and experienced by the person being reinforced. We often see clients who tend to rush from their ambition to an Action Step to progress without giving time or eye contact for reinforcement to occur. This not only means the reinforcement is ineffective but also it is punishing for other group members who are practicing their reinforcement and "reading the room" skills. If clients are not attending to others and missing potential reinforcement in skills group, it is likely they are doing this at work or school, with family, and in other important relationships, and these individuals are also being punished for attempts to reinforce. Therefore, the group leaders should stop the client if they are moving through the Check-In without looking up or attending to other group members and coach them to effectively notice and accept reinforcement from the group (which also reinforces group members for being reinforcing). Self-invalidation should be blocked.

iv. After reporting the parts of the Action Step they did complete, the client reports on the parts of it they did not complete, if any.

f. *Effective Behavior*

i. The Check-In form asks clients to list one effective thing they did to complete their Action Step. Unless the client completed absolutely no part of their Action Step, they should be asked to report on what they did accomplish. The client's description of this effective thing should not just repeat their progress report—the key is *how* the progress was made.

ii. Clients may try and say they didn't do anything effective, but this behavior should be blocked. The group may need to help the client identify a skill or strategy they used.

iii. The goal here is to highlight for the group each week effective ways to achieve Action Steps and ambitions. This reinforces the idea that progress does not miraculously or haphazardly happen, but instead is a direct result of their own behavior.

iv. Leaders should try to highlight categories illustrated by clients' shared effective behavior. This helps clients to learn from each other's examples, as well as their own (see the Examples of Effective Behaviors and Ways to Prevent Avoidance handout in the "DBT Next Steps Skills Overview" section of the *DBT Next Steps Skills Handouts* volume). For instance:

- Scheduling
- Doing it right away
- Keeping mindful of your Action Step
- Keeping mindful of your ambition
- Taking advantage of opportunities that arise
- Using the contingency of having to report to the group as a deadline
- Anticipating positive reinforcement from the group
- Using opposite action

v. These are the skills and strategies they need to learn to keep going and build on past effective pieces as well as to troubleshoot when they get stuck.

g. *Avoidance*

i. As above, clients are also asked to identify ways they avoided completing their Action Step. Avoidance in DBT Next Steps is not meant to imply intention or moral failing. It simply means that a behavior interfered with progress this week, whether or not this was intended or something of which the client was aware. Like identifying effective steps, clients should not repeat their lack of progress as their avoidant behavior, and instead identify ineffective behaviors associated with that lack of progress.

ii. In explaining this to clients, one might say, "When you first came to DBT, the ways you avoided were probably pretty obvious: You decided not to come to session, you didn't get out of bed, you didn't do the homework, you quit rather than finding a solution. To get into DBT Next Steps, you have learned skills to be effective and you are no longer doing clear avoidance behaviors. What is getting in your way now is often a lot more subtle and harder to see. Our job in DBT Next Steps is to find all the small, sneaky ways your brain has to avoid things that it doesn't want to do, like deciding other things are more important, or forgetting, or procrastinating."

iii. Avoidance in DBT Next Steps Check-In only applies if the Action or Employment Step was not completed by the beginning of group. If the Action Step was completed right before group after procrastinating all week, this is not defined as avoidance in this context. Instead, it is described as "using a deadline," which is effective and normative.

iv. Again, it's important to help clients categorize avoidance into larger categories to which they can become more and more alert (again, see the Examples of Effective Behaviors and Ways to Prevent Avoidance handout in the "DBT Next Steps Overview" section of *DBT Next Steps Skills Handouts*):

- Forgetting
- Willfulness
- Prioritizing other things
- Giving in to anxiety
- Getting disorganized and not having time
- Procrastinating
- Telling yourself it isn't that important
- Forgetting or losing touch with the importance of the ambition

v. The goal is for the clients to hear themselves and others in the group talking about avoidance repeatedly until they have over-learned the concept and can catch themselves when having urges to avoid before actually avoiding.

vi. We want clients to learn that Action Steps and ambitions aren't missed because of a fatal flaw or other global failure of a person, but rather by a series of small behaviors that add up to avoidance. Avoidance will make more and more sense to the clients, eventually feeling less personal and devastating and much easier to solve and troubleshoot.

h. *Preventing Avoidance*

   i. Asking clients to identify how they will prevent avoidance in the future serves multiple purposes. It is a chance to apply the knowledge of effective versus avoidance behaviors in future planning. It helps if other clients chip in as they may see the situation more objectively; it is also excellent practice for them in a less personal situation. Considering how to prevent avoidance also teaches troubleshooting, which is a critical skill if these clients are to become self-sufficient.

   ii. As noted by the double asterisks (**) on the form, this is a good place for other clients to generate possible solutions. Skills leaders may need to go back to the client for a commitment to one or two of the solutions generated by the group, or the discussion may become too diffuse to be useful. Asking the client to choose from group-generated solutions also models making a choice and a commitment in a systematic way.

   iii. Block attempts to use "willpower" or "wishful thinking" as strategies here (e.g., "I just won't do that next week"). That would be an example of self-invalidation and oversimplifying the ease of solving the problem. Coach the client and the group to come up with specific, mindful, and concrete steps the individual can take that will realistically block this avoidance behavior in the future (at least somewhat, if shaping is needed). Remember that letting clients use willpower teaches that willpower and wishful thinking are effective strategies you hope they will use more in the future, and reinforces irritated, shy, or other mood-dependent behaviors as reasons to stop troubleshooting—something else you probably don't want to reinforce!

i. *Emotion*

   i. Clients are asked to observe emotion(s) they experienced while working on their Action Steps. This doesn't mean that the emotion was caused by their Action Steps—it could be that the emotion was going on for other reasons (e.g., background sadness, anger at a therapist).

   ii. The purpose of identifying an emotion is to have clients become more aware of the emotions they experience and how they relate to the Action Steps and progress. This also promotes an emotion focus in group, which is an important part of DBT.

   iii. Typically, as clients move through the modules of skills-training group, they are more and more likely to identify joy, pride, contentment, and happiness in relation to their Action Steps and ambitions (as opposed to the anger, frustration, shame, and sadness they associate with ambitions early in DBT Next Steps group). It is helpful for other clients to see the positive emotions with which the Action Steps and ambitions are associated in senior clients and for those feeling positive emotions to recognize and celebrate that fact.

j. *Generating a New Target*

   i. Following a review of the previous Action Step and progress, the client is asked to generate a new target. The purpose is to develop an Action Step that is challenging, relevant to their goal, and shows a high likelihood of success.

ii. Following the contingency management principles in Chapter 7 and didactics principles in Chapter 9, as well as the shaping rules in Chapter 2 of *Don't Shoot the Dog* (Pryor, 2018), is key here, as clients are essentially being taught to shape their own behavior toward their ambitions.

iii. Two key rules:

- Follow the guidance on Action Steps (see 3c above).
- Be sure that the client is reinforcing and being reinforced for their work on their Action Steps (see 3e above) and not being invalidated by themselves or others. The reinforcement of the group is too far away from the behavior to compete with the immediacy of negative self-talk or invalidation in the client's day-to-day environment.

iv. Clients sometimes want to have more than one Action or Employment Step. They can have as many as three or four if they are clearly related and they have a 50% chance of doing all of them. Action Steps are not their to-do list of everything they have to get done; this is an exercise in carefully crafting a task such that success is inevitable.

v. New Action and Employment Steps need to be stated concisely and specifically (see 3c above) and written down by the client and the skills co-leader.

vi. As noted by the ** on the form, this is a good place for other clients to actively participate, as they learn as much by assisting someone else (where they can be more objective) as by going through the process themselves. The leader may need to broker this discussion and help the client choose the next Action and Employment Steps using commitment strategies. It is important to orient clients to the dialectics of giving suggestions and feedback to each other. On the one hand, it's a great learning experience for them and they may understand the issues that another client faces more than the skills leaders. On the other hand, sometimes a client really wants feedback from the skills leader more than other clients. It is an opportunity for other clients to practice "reading the room" and deciding when to speak up and when not to.

Review of Assignments

1. After Check-In, the skills leaders review how the clients did on their assignments from last week.
2. In DBT Next Steps, all assignments are completed in writing. There are several reasons for this. First, the material moves very quickly and is reviewed only once, so it is important the clients gain as full an understanding of the material as possible. Second, one goal of the DBT Next Steps Skills Curriculum is to create a skills notebook that can be used as a reference in the years ahead. Many assignments without any notes on them would not be sufficient to understand years later when they are needed, so having each written, complete assignment provides a model of how to use that skill or strategy. Finally, DBT Next Steps is modeled on business meetings and college classes in which assignments are expected to be complete and generally written. Being able to have detailed (but not too detailed), cogent, legible, and comprehensive assignments is an important skill that requires steady practice to achieve. Therefore, it is critical that it become a habit in DBT Next Steps.

3. When the review of assignments starts, the skills leader reminds everyone of the page number of the assignment from last week (or asks a client to do so) and turns to that page. Clients who do not follow the nonverbal cue should be prompted to move to that page. In some cases, some irreverence here is helpful to highlight that not following that cue is problematic (e.g., "Sheila, you with us?" or "I'm not thinking, Ken, that I actually have to tell you to go to page *X*, do I?" or, if it was a large part of the group, "Hey . . . this wouldn't be cool at work or school would it—that you were directed to the assignment and you just sat there?").
4. Next, the skills leader asks who has completed all parts of the assignment from last week. Both the skills leader and co-leader should look around the table to see that everyone has done the assignment in writing. Remind clients who have not completed it in writing that they need to do so and have it reviewed by the skills co-leader as soon as possible (e.g., "You are going to get that done in writing and review with Mike next week, right?" or "It is important that your notebook is complete so you can use it as a reference in years to come. Be sure to write down what you did and review it with Jenna, OK?").
5. Once a norm of completed homework gets set, then you should *not* ask if everyone has done it, as that is not normative in the work or school world. In this case, the skills leader should proceed as if everyone has completed the assignment, and the skills leader or co-leader can remark on those clients who haven't.
6. It is important to reinforce thorough completion of assignments as well as new insights, ambitious or creative assignments or otherwise going beyond the requirements, clients being ready to present their assignments, and being flexible about how they are asked to present their work.
7. Some clients will overdo their assignments or be perfectionistic about them. Do NOT reinforce this behavior as it is often the reason they have not succeeded at work, school, self-management, or social relationships. Differentially reinforce effective behavior and highlight ways that perfectionism interfered or how they went too far. Use level 4 validation to confirm that they have good reason to do this while simultaneously highlighting it as ineffective. For example, the skills leader could say:

   > "Given that your parents were always critical or asking for more, it is understandable that you think you need to do more than the assignment asks for. However, bosses and teachers don't want to review more work than they have to and value getting exactly what they asked for over getting more. DBT Next Steps is a good opportunity to calibrate yourself to people more typical than your parents. So, this part where you did what was asked is great. And, next time, don't add more work than has been requested or check with me first."

8. If a client repeatedly doesn't complete their homework or needs reminding about it, this should be highlighted individually by the leader or co-leader before or after group or by phone. Clients should be reminded of the professional behavior expected in DBT Next Steps and encouraged to work on this with their individual therapist immediately.
9. Clients cannot have four or more assignments incomplete at any time during DBT Next Steps without being suspended from group until they have done them. As noted above, co-leaders need to track whether homework is completed and alert clients if concerned that they are four assignments behind. Clients are expected to be able to determine this

themselves by paging through the modules they have completed so far and seeing how many of them are not filled in completely. If a skills co-leader believes someone might be too far behind, the client needs to show the skills leader that their book is complete to within four assignments in order to continue in group.

10. Clients are responsible for bringing completed assignments to the skills co-leader's attention before group, during break, or after group. Skills co-leaders should review for completeness and general accuracy. If time allows, it is best if the skills co-leader reviews assignments in detail and provides feedback; however, this is often not possible.
11. Clients practice professional social skills in reviewing their homework with the skills co-leader (e.g., proactively seeking out the skills co-leader, not asking to show the co-leader their assignments during group, assuring that the co-leader has sufficient time to review an assignment at that moment, not showing an assignment half completed, not showing anything to the skills leader unless that leader is running group alone that day or there is another good reason to do so). Clients should use the Practice Professional Behavior in DBT Next Steps handout from *DBT Next Steps Skills Handouts* volume as described above. If their behavior is not professional, the client should be prompted to stop now and restart again more skillfully at the appropriate time.
12. DBT Next Steps skills group time is generally insufficient for each client to review their assignment in the detail that is common in SDBT. Having the assignments in writing means less review is required and that review of assignments moves quickly. The teaching lesson plans in the subsequent chapters also provide tips that will help in reviewing the homework efficiently. DBT Next Steps clients are expected to pay sufficient attention and take sufficient notes to ensure that their assignments are correctly completed without individual attention being necessary. That is how this often occurs in work and school settings. When a client is not able to do this—in general or for a particular assignment or module that is difficult for them—the client should bring the assignment to individual therapy for further discussion to ensure their mastery of the material.

Review of New Material

1. DBT Next Steps groups end with teaching the new material for that week. Because of the time it will take for all the other steps of the DBT Next Steps skills-training group to be covered, there is generally going to be, at best, 30 minutes left to teach new material and, at worst, 15–20 minutes. This is to be expected, and a dialectical balance must be struck to try to devote as much time as possible to new teaching without rushing Good News, Check-In, or the review of assignments so much that they lose their value. This balance takes practice and coordination between the leader and co-leader.
2. Some new material can be taught very quickly so time is less relevant. Some material is best understood by clients through the review of assignments after they have attempted it. In those cases, give the clients the skeleton teaching and then plan more time for the review of assignments the next week.
3. Teaching new material should be done as you would in a business meeting or college class. This is not different from what occurred in the other sections of DBT Next Steps groups, but

is particularly important to give clients relevant experience with professional settings and help them learn how to keep up, stay focused, and the like on their own without prompting from the co-leader, as is typical in an SDBT group. Similar expectations apply to skills leaders as to clients to be professional, not fragilize the clients, and understand the material fully.

4. Clients should be directed at the beginning (or reminded when new clients join) that we expect them to take notes. As with the review of assignments, we want the skills notebook to include sufficient notes so that clients can understand the material if they go back to it years later. If clients don't believe they need to take notes, then they should be instructed to engage in other behaviors that convince the skills leader and co-leader of their undivided attention and comprehension of the material, such as removing other distractions, making eye contact, demonstrating they are comprehending the material through their comments and questions, and doing the homework correctly. If they are not able to do these things, they should be redirected to taking notes or using other tools to be sure they understand the material fully. As with everything else in DBT Next Steps, clients should ask questions in a professional manner and demonstrate their interest in the answers.
5. Clients' professional behavior, interest, and attention should be reinforced by skills leaders and co-leaders. Using the principles of reinforcement, such behaviors should be reinforced continuously until established and then intermittently. At first, leaders and co-leaders should discuss how they want to manage these contingencies ahead of time so they can track what they are reinforcing and how often. Over time, this becomes second nature.
6. Statements of helplessness, general noncomprehension, fragility, hopelessness, and so forth should NOT be reinforced. Irreverent comments ("You wouldn't say that at school, would you?"; or "That is not a professional thing to say—I don't recommend you say that at work. Please talk with your therapist about it and don't say it here"; or "That is not a great way to sell yourself to a new friend") should be used to prompt more effective behavior. Persistent behavior should be highlighted by the skills leader or co-leader at break, before or after group, or by phone or letter. Clients should be encouraged to seek assistance from their individual therapist to be more effective during group.

Closing of Group Session

1. There is no specific closing of DBT Next Steps group sessions. This is an opportunity for clients to end effectively without special reminders about completing their Check-In and assignments. They should follow the professional behavior guidelines outlined in the "DBT Next Steps Overview" section of the *DBT Next Steps Skills Handouts* volume and "read the room" as discussed above.
2. If clients are not following professional behavior guidelines, it is important that this be addressed right away.
   a. If it is one person, they should be pulled aside or receive a call from a group leader later to describe the problem and ask for it to be resolved. Group leaders should handle this as much as possible like a supervisor or boss would. If the client becomes defensive, coach professional behavior and GIVE skills. If this is not quickly resolved, the individual therapist should take over as with any other TIB.

b. If the entire group is having an issue, highlight this as the clients are leaving using a brief comment or joke (as a supervisor might), but don't delay ending group. If the behavior persists, highlight it again and then take a brief time at the beginning of the next group to describe the problem and a potential solution, and ask for commitment and troubleshooting. If a single client is a holdout on finding a solution, then go to 2a above to address the matter as an individual issue.

Session-by-Session Lesson Plans

The following chapters give the lesson plans specific to each skill in the *DBT Next Steps Skills Handouts* volume. Each of the six modules starts with some "General Notes." Then weeks 1–4 of each module are described in detail. First, "Key Points for Teaching" describes how to teach that day's skills. Second, "Presenting the Assignment" provides guidance for how to orient to the assigned task the clients will be completing during the week. Finally, "Review the Assignment" offers guidance on points to consider or address at the beginning of the next week's class, including what to assess and what to reinforce.

CHAPTER 15

Module: Perfectionism versus Reinforcement

General Notes

1. The focus of this module is the Self-Management Recovery Goals:
   - Have an effective method for managing your monthly budget and one-time expenses (e.g., new tires) so you stay within your income.
   - Have sufficient emergency fund savings to cover 3 months of living expenses in case you lose your job.
   - Have an effective method of savings for things you would enjoy.
   - Have an effective method for getting out of debt/reducing debt to a reasonable level.
   - Have an effective method for managing your time in line with your Wise Mind values.
   - Have an effective method for managing your time that gets key things done on schedule.
   - Have an effective method for managing your time that balances work, leisure, household, and downtime.
   - Have an effective method of preventing illness and psychiatric symptoms from impacting your functioning.
   - Have an effective method of managing chronic illness or pain to minimize its impact on your quality of life.
2. If clients are to achieve these goals, they absolutely need to break through perfectionistic patterns and use effective positive reinforcement tools—which are the focus of the module.
3. This is a module where the client needs to engage the individual therapist. As the therapist may be focused on other topics, it is helpful to alert the client that they should DEAR MAN their therapist for time to discuss their assignments in this module and orient the therapist that there are DBT Next Steps assignments to review.

4. It is not possible to do more than overview the principles of reinforcement in this module during skills training. If the Self-Management Recovery Goals are an important target in DBT Next Steps for a particular client (which they usually are), then the client will also need to:
   a. Read the book *Don't Shoot the Dog* (Pryor, 2018) or listen to the "Hidden Brain" podcast about it (Schmidt et al., 2018) and search for "clicker training videos" online. These are optional assignments because we have found that DBT Next Steps group leaders do not always assign the reading and that some clients don't do it. It is a dialectic, and as a synthesis, we have included the material as optional.
   b. The individual therapist will need to really take this material on in individual therapy if they want their client to be able to implement it accurately, effectively, and consistently in a follow-up to this module. The majority of clients simply can't both learn and use this material without substantial coaching beyond the 2 weeks on alternatives to perfectionism and 2 weeks on behavioral strategies taught in DBT Next Steps skills group.

Week 1: Perfectionism versus High Achievement

Key Points for Teaching

1. Perfectionism is used as an example of the epitome of losing a dialectic because:
   a. It is so prevalent among DBT clients.
   b. It is associated with poor outcomes in psychotherapy.
2. Consider briefly re-orienting to the aspect of biosocial theory where the invalidating environment oversimplifies the ease of problem solving. It often is the case that individuals raised in such an invalidating environment will self-invalidate by setting unreasonable and unattainable goals.
   a. Such an invalidating environment does not model distress tolerance or the skills needed to problem-solve to achieve a goal.
   b. Engage the group in considering how perfectionism might develop from this learning history. (If this conversation will take over the discussion, given the group makeup, then you can skip this discussion and just make a teaching point.)
3. Review the characteristics of perfectionism (pp. 21–22 of *DBT Next Steps Skills Handouts*) to help clients understand what perfectionism is and isn't and how it applies to their life.
   a. Go around the room having clients read aloud each characteristic. Ask the rest of the clients to raise their hand and check the box if it applies to them. As a group, generate examples, particularly of how this arises in different contexts (e.g., perfectionism showing up while writing emails, being available to a friend, preparing meals).
   b. Discuss the pros and cons of perfectionism. Highlighting the cons, increase client commitment to stop perfectionism wherever they can.
4. Using the handout One Middle Road: High Achievement (p. 23), help clients understand how high achievement and healthy striving are not perfectionism.
   a. As with perfectionism characteristics, go around the room having clients read aloud each one. Ask the rest of the clients to raise their hand if it applies to them. As a group, generate examples—this will be difficult for many clients.

b. Discuss the pros and cons of high achieving instead of perfectionism. Highlighting the pros, increase client commitment to being a high achiever wherever they can.

Presenting the Week 1 Assignment

1. Orient to the Week 1 Assignment: Exploring High Achievement over Perfectionism (pp. 24–26), which has seven steps and involves daily practice as well as an interview with the therapist. (Unless it would fragilize your particular group members, you may want to highlight that this means they have to start the assignment by the next day.)
2. It is important to highlight that you expect them to complete the entire assignment. For instance, Question 2 asks the clients to do an analysis of pros and cons where the effective behavior is being a high achiever and the undesirable behavior is being a perfectionist. After identifying the pros and cons of each, the next page then asks clients to relist the pros of being a high achiever alongside the cons of perfectionism (i.e., selectively copying from the previous page). Clients often skip this list, but it is the one you really want them to keep and refer to.
3. Emphasize that giving yourself credit for small accomplishments (see Question 3 on the assignment sheet) involves being mindful of small, minor, less significant moments of effectiveness that might be easily overlooked by a perfectionist mindset. Mindfulness here involves both noticing and describing what you notice without judgment.
4. For Questions 4 and 5—examples of past mistakes and radical acceptance statements—highlight this as a good place to incorporate middle path and loving kindness strategies.

Reviewing the Week 1 Assignment

1. We have found it most effective to review each of the seven steps for the whole group before moving to the next. That is, review Step 1 for everyone, then Step 2 for everyone, and so on.
2. For Question 2, make sure the clients have written out their list of the pros of high achieving and cons of perfectionism and taken a photo or saved their list in a handy location. You might ask how they intend to remember to check the list when they need to.
3. For Question 3, we often go around the room a few times, with clients indicating their small achievements. It can be helpful to remind everyone what self-invalidation looks like before you start, and if anyone self-invalidates as they read their achievement, group members can practice making a kind observation and that person can reread their achievement without any self-invalidation.
4. For Question 5, highlight if someone wrote an approval rather than acceptance statement. Ask them to try and revise their statement so it reflects what they radically accept as true about themself without the positive judgment.
5. When reviewing "giving permission to make mistakes" (Question 6), have everyone say their sentence out loud in group. Be sure to reinforce their conviction and participation in reading the sentence and how they practiced it. Of course, if they don't say it with conviction, the group leaders and/or members can kindly observe this and ask them to try again. You want to rehearse effective, not ineffective, behavior and end on a high note.
6. For Question 7, ask for a show of hands or nods if clients did answer it. Then ask the group

as a whole for any observations they might have about their discussion with their therapist. (Best not to go one by one here as some clients will not want to share details about this discussion.)

Week 2: Another Middle Road Option: Being Average

Key Points for Teaching

1. The goal is to up the ante with the clients to get them to not only replace perfectionism with high achievement (a change in perspective that is consistent with achievement) but also with being average (which is not).
2. The idea of being average generally is a very uncomfortable and sometimes unpleasant idea to DBT Next Steps clients.
3. Review the bell curve on the handout to illustrate an average person as the peak in the middle, not the smaller number of people at the high or lower ends.
4. Using the Week 2: Another Middle Road Option: Being Average handout (p. 27), have a discussion about average differing from "bad," the advantages of being average, and the ways being average can increase their overall chances of success.
5. Not all behaviors need to be high achieving, and high achievement in some areas is facilitated by being average in others. Group leaders can provide modeling of the helpful choices that can be made (e.g., some people who are ambitious at work choose to be average housekeepers; some people who excel at a healthy diet and exercise choose to drive when they are short on time, even though high achievement by their values is to take the bus, bike, or walk).
6. It can also be helpful to clarify that the context in which they are high achieving or being average will naturally shift over time and with certain challenges (e.g., when they get sick, they may have to become average at work and a high achiever at rest to get well faster).
7. Increase clients' commitment to being average in some areas as part of seeing the whole picture and strategizing effectively to reach their personal goals.

Presenting the Week 2 Assignment

1. The Week 2 Assignment: Practicing Alternatives to Being a Perfectionist (pp. 28–32) asks clients to replace perfectionist behavior with both high achievement and being average.
2. The goal of Question 1 is brainstorming, so encourage a long, mindful, and creative list.
3. Clients are then asked to select two examples of behaviors listed in the response to Question 1 to address for the week. Encourage them to pick small perfectionist behaviors to which they aren't too attached (especially since they will have only 1 week to work on this). If a client is feeling willful about changing a perfectionist behavior at all, they will avoid the assignment, rather than fully practice the strategies surrounding it.
4. For Behavior 1, they will be practicing high-achiever strategies, and for Behavior 2, they will practice being average.

5. The key to learning here is not that they succeed at their high-achieving and being average alternatives, per se, but that they practice the strategies suggested and observe what each is like, and compare and contrast them.
6. Remind clients to reduce perfectionism about doing this assignment itself and instead take a high-achieving (rather than average, in this case) approach.
7. Ask them to keep their eyes on the prize of experiencing a different way of being, rather than making a permanent life change. A critical part of this homework is practicing the skill of stepping back and observing your own behavior and experience.
8. For Question 3a, be sure the clients understand that they need to take Behavior 1 and replace it with a high-achieving alternative (going back to p. 23 for examples to work from). The high-achieving alternative needs to be refined to match and replace Behavior 1, rather than their just trying to be high achieving in general. This first step is a thought exercise concerning what a good substitute might be, and it can be done during group if there is time, or the leaders can model taking one of their perfectionist behaviors and replacing it with a high-achieving one with advice from the group.
    - *Example 1:* As part of Question 1 of the Week 2 Assignment (p. 28), based on reviewing the lists of perfectionist characteristics as well as her homework, an adolescent identifies that she ruminates for hours if she makes any kind of mistake and avoids doing things for fear of making mistakes. For Question 2, she could make ruminating about mistakes Perfectionist Behavior 1 and discounting positive feedback Perfectionist Behavior 2. With the group's help on her response to Question 3a, she could replace rumination about mistakes (Perfectionist Behavior 1) with a high-achieving alternative, such as describing what she did well in the situation and then distracting herself so she doesn't return to rumination.
    - *Example 2:* Based on reviewing the lists of perfectionist characteristics as well as his homework, an adult client who wants to be a restaurant cook identifies that he has all-or-nothing thinking and that he overemphasizes "shoulds" and has a lot of "right ways" things have to be done at work that take longer than the time he has in a busy restaurant kitchen. For Question 2, he could make all-or-nothing thinking Perfectionist Behavior 1 and overemphasizing "shoulds" as Perfectionist Behavior 2. With the group's help on his response to Question 3a, he could replace all-or-nothing thinking about his career (Perfectionist Behavior 1) with a high-achieving alternative, such as using the Cope Ahead skill to visualize his career progress as a series of steps toward his goal of being a cook in the kind of restaurant he aspires to work in and then to each day imagine those steps when he has all-or-nothing thoughts.
9. Question 3b involves putting Question 3a into practice during the week and writing down your observations.
10. For Question 3c, make sure the clients understand that they are not continuing to work on Behavior 1 and are instead moving on to Perfectionist Behavior 2 (p. 31). Again, the first step (in responding to Question 3c) is a thought exercise concerning what being average is and how you could practice that in group; the response to Question 3d means putting this into practice during the week and observing.
    - *Example 1:* For Question 3c, the adolescent above could decide to replace avoiding doing things for fear of making mistakes (Perfectionist Behavior 2) with an average behavior,

such as doing one thing a day with a reasonable chance of making a mistake in a situation where this won't be a serious issue. For instance, not running the spellchecker on an assignment for a teacher who isn't overly concerned about spelling or messaging a friend about something unimportant and not reading over your email or text before hitting send.

- *Example 2:* For Question 3c, the adult above could decide to replace overemphasizing "shoulds" at work (Perfectionist Behavior 2) with an average behavior, such as when you can imagine a more efficient way to do something, simply letting it pass, and allowing others to be the leader, with you just following along. For instance, he could use Wise Mind to pick two tasks at his job where the boss says it has to be done a certain way, but almost no one ever does it that way and it really doesn't seem to matter. He could then practice doing the task the way others do it, instead of falling behind because he was doing it the "right" way.

11. Question 4 (p. 32) is a separate part of the assignment, not a follow-through on Questions 1–3. The goal is to fully participate on a single day—just 1 day during the week. Help the group understand what expectations are and how such expectations can prevent you from fully experiencing your life. Perhaps have the group practice imagining how their morning begins and what happens as they go through the first hour or 2 of their day. Ask clients to share the first expectation that comes into their mind. Coach them to let go of that expectation and return to imagining their day moving forward. Then another group member can note the first expectation they noticed, and so on. If something isn't really an expectation, then clarify and shape that for the clients. Then ask them to practice this in real life—pick 1 day over the next week to watch for any expectation; when one flashes through their mind, ask them to let go of it and return to having no expectations.
12. As with many other DBT Next Steps assignments, this final step is designed to give clients a particular experience, rather than asking them to live the rest of their life without expectations. Some clients will choose to start doing this exercise all the time, but that isn't the point of the assignment and is up to them and their individual therapist. (Could actually be an example of perfectionism!)

Reviewing the Week 2 Assignment

1. Ask each member to reflect on their experience of replacing their perfectionistic behaviors with something more effective—with a high-achieving and average alternative. Did anything surprise them? Did they have preferences for high-achieving vs. average strategies? With this experience under their belt, in the future, where might they choose to apply high-achieving strategies and where might being average be more effective?
2. Ask the group to volunteer things they noticed themselves expecting. (You don't have to go around the room—just have clients call out their experiences.)
3. Then ask each person to observe their experience of not expecting anything. During the observations, ask them to notice how this experience was different from their typical life. Were there some surprises? Did they prefer not having expectations, or did they prefer having them? Did they notice behaving or feeling differently than they do on days where they have expectations?
4. The group leader's focus should be on reinforcing creativity, courage, participation, persistence, and flexibility.

Week 3: The Basics of Reinforcement

Key Points for Teaching

1. This month's module teaches reinforcement principles based on the book *Don't Shoot the Dog* (Pryor, 2018). This is a self-help manual that teaches how to use positive reinforcement to improve your own and others' behavior. The reading is optional and highly encouraged. It is relatively easy to read and applies many animal-training concepts to people and self-help. Used copies of the book are generally inexpensive or available at the library, or your program might want to keep some copies on hand for clients to borrow.
2. It is especially critical for effective teaching of this module that the skills-training leaders have read *Don't Shoot the Dog* and practiced the DBT Next Steps homework exercises themselves until they are successful. If the leaders have not experienced the power of reinforcement to change their own stubborn behaviors and those of at least one other person in their lives, it is not feasible to teach this module. Possible behaviors for skills leaders to try and change with reinforcement are exercising, eating, sleeping, on-time charting, lateness, getting your partner to cook more often, getting your partner to drive more safely, getting your kids to pick up after themselves, getting your dog to not bark at the door, and the like.
3. If DBT Next Steps clinicians do not have a solid understanding of behavioral principles and how to apply them, the team might consider spending time doing a study group based on *Don't Shoot the Dog* or *Self-Management: Using Behavioral and Cognitive Principles to Manage Your Life* by Edward P. Sarafino (2011). The latter is a college textbook that has students pick a behavior they want to change to achieve a goal. Each chapter then teaches a CBT principle; the homework is to apply the principle to the behavior you are trying to change. When we did this as part of our DBT consultation team, members read each chapter on their own, and we spent the first 30 minutes of the meeting reviewing our homework from the previous chapter and committing to doing the next chapter the following week. As a slower alternative, the team could take a chapter a month and dedicate part of one team/month to this. Don't ask most clients to read *Self-Management*, as *Don't Shoot the Dog* is more effective for the lay public.
4. It can be very uncomfortable for some clients to think about deliberately changing others' behavior using reinforcement—it can seem underhanded, especially as most reinforcement of others won't work if you tell them you are doing it. The important message for the clients to understand is that reinforcement and punishment of others' behavior are inevitable—there is no way to stop them from happening—and the point is to get more effective at doing so. A good illustration is to explain which of your own behaviors the clients' behavior in the group has reinforced and punished, and how you would appreciate them reinforcing you for the behaviors you do engage in that help them—for example, "You have told me it helps you learn if I say things more simply and directly. If you all can figure out what is reinforcing to me, then you can reinforce me when I say things simply and directly. That would be awesome!" What is reinforcing depends on the skills leader, of course, but examples might be smiling, eye contact, validation, sharing what they think the leader is saying to show they understand.
5. Reinforcing someone for doing something that makes them proud or happy is probably not going to be a problem, whereas reinforcing someone for doing what you want that is

not in their best interest is experienced as manipulation. That is, don't "con" people: Don't reinforce them for eating unhealthy food when they are on a diet or going to a drinking establishment if they are sober, and don't get them to cut school or pay your bills. While this might work from a DEAR MAN objective, it will likely damage your relationship and your self-respect.

6. Another important note is that what a client might think is reinforcing to someone—such as smiling or giving them gifts or compliments—may not actually be reinforcing to that person. Learning what is truly reinforcing to someone else and providing that reinforcement when they do something good for your relationship are helpful to the relationship and make it more enjoyable and positive for both parties. Give examples where people are trying to use reinforcement with someone but choose the wrong reinforcers. Highlight how the behavior they wanted was actually suppressed (i.e., punished) and that the person did less of what was wanted and not more. (For example, if someone thinks they are reinforcing with eye contact when an older person is talking, but the older person is from a culture where direct eye contact from a younger person is considered insulting, it will not be reinforcing to them.)
7. A theme throughout DBT Next Steps is learning to "read a room" and using observe and describe skills to learn other people's reinforcers. An important DBT Next Steps goal is for clients to learn how to determine reinforcers by observation without having to ask explicitly. This will allow them to be significantly more effective in work, school, and social situations. This theme is tackled explicitly in this module and should be highlighted throughout the DBT Next Steps program in both skills-training group and individual therapy.
8. The Week 3: The Basics of Reinforcement handout (pp. 33–36) walks clients through key points of behaviorism covered in *Don't Shoot the Dog*, followed by an in-class practice example (Practicing Reinforcement, p. 37). The in-class example can be one person's example that everyone works through (potentially the group leader, who can illustrate the teaching points with their description), or each person can simply work through their own example.
9. Discuss the difference between reinforcement and reward, and how reinforcers are not always obvious. Highlight examples where seeming rewards are actually not reinforcing. For instance, some people would not like to see their picture on the wall as employee of the month, or they may not want the free parking space that comes with being named employee of the year if they don't have a car.
10. Highlight that when we (or Karen Pryor) say that the subject is "learning what the trainer wants" or "understands what is wanted," we are not saying that someone knows this intellectually or in their frontal lobe (Pryor, 2018). This kind of learning is something more instinctive than that based in the brainstem (a.k.a. "lizard brain"). The mind makes these connections largely at an unconscious level, and that is the way it is meant to work. There is no need to explain intellectually what you want the person to learn behaviorally. In fact, sometimes doing that interferes (e.g., your spouse may learn to take out the trash unconsciously through reinforcement and would actively balk at taking out the trash if you intellectually explained that you would be reinforcing them to do so).
11. Discuss the difference between positive and negative reinforcement and between negative

reinforcement and punishment. Especially important is the concept that punishment comes after a behavior and cannot be controlled by a change in that behavior, where negative reinforcement works because of immediate withdrawal of the aversive stimuli as soon as the desired behavior occurs. The example from *Don't Shoot the Dog* is the aunt who frowns disapprovingly when you put your feet on her coffee table, and then relaxes and smiles again when you take your feet off it. If she just frowned the rest of visit, that would be punishment. Removing the negative when you change is negative reinforcement and helps you learn specifically what is wanted.

12. Positive reinforcement is the most desirable reinforcer for the clients to use for two reasons. First, it is simpler and easier to pull off without mistakes. Second, it is more relationship building than negative reinforcement, which may involve adding an aversive so you can then remove it as the reinforcement. Adding aversives is tricky and more likely to cause bad feelings. As noted in Chapter 4 ("Untraining") in *Don't Shoot the Dog*, negative reinforcement works most effectively when the person intellectually agrees that the behavior should occur (e.g., most kids are fine with being nagged to do their homework Sunday afternoon or evening, but would resent and push back against being nagged—the negative reinforcer—on Friday night).
13. Another crucial point is that you can only determine if your behavior is reinforcing or not by whether the subject's behavior increases. It is irrelevant how reinforcing the trainer thinks or believes something is. If the subject's behavior does not increase when that reinforcer is provided immediately after the behavior, it isn't serving as a reinforcer.
14. Discuss how crucial timing is. Reinforcement provided too late is most likely reinforcing something irrelevant to the behavior you were trying to reinforce. That is, you ignored the behavior at the time and whatever the subject was doing later when you provided the reinforcer is what will be reinforced. In *Don't Shoot the Dog*, reinforcing soccer kicks in the locker room after the game reinforces being with the team or being around the coach, yet is unlikely to reinforce the specific kick. This is why coaches run up and down the field giving feedback during the game.
15. You may want to highlight that the trainer should not use reinforcers (including aversives to remove for negative reinforcement) that are aversive to the trainer. If so, the trainer will not be reinforced to follow the system and, in fact, will work to avoid it. Parents make this mistake by grounding a kid such that the kid is around the house in a bad mood or they have to structure their life around policing the grounding, which they eventually tire of and give up as a consequence. Thus, negative reinforcement (withdrawing the grounding) either comes in response to a kid's bad mood (i.e., the kid's mood is really annoying and functionally nagging the parents, so they remove the grounding to make it go away) or is irrelevant to the kid's behavior (i.e., grounding stops because of their fatigue, rather than the kid's behavior improving), so nothing useful is learned.
16. You may want to highlight that big reinforcers can be problematic. They both get used up too quickly and take too long to enjoy before the subject is interested in more. They can also be expensive or unrealistic, which can be aversive to the trainer, who will therefore work to avoid having to give it. You want to use the smallest reinforcer that will work and can use a sum of these to build to a big reinforcer (e.g., 10 gold stars = 1 latte). This is also known as a

"contingency management" or "token economy" system. Surprisingly, if you have a calendar to which you are adding gold stars or use a gold star app on your phone, you may find the stars themselves are reinforcing and you don't need the big reinforcer.

17. Reinforcers should be distinct. If you use a reinforcer that you provide at other times, you'll also be reinforcing no behavior or problem behaviors. This will confuse the subject, and they won't learn what behavior is being reinforced. Reinforcement is information about what you want, and if you say you want things when you don't, the subject won't be able to learn when to produce them. For example, if you give your child a food they like when they are tired and cranky, you might want to avoid using that as a reinforcer at other times because you'll be inadvertently reinforcing when they are cranky as well and they may not understand what you want.
18. Discuss when to tell a subject that you are reinforcing them. Often being told they are being reinforced makes the reinforcers aversive, and the subject will be reinforced by you stopping what you think are reinforcers rather than providing them. For example, telling your spouse that you are putting them on a reinforcement program to get them to clean the house may be offensive to them, so any praise, appreciation, or validation you were offering as reinforcement becomes punishing if it refers to cleaning the house. In fact, they will be reinforced by you giving up—that is, no longer reinforcing cleaning the house. Now they aren't cleaning the house any more than before, and to them cleaning the house may become a hot-button topic so it may actually become more difficult to get them to change than before. On the other hand, there are times when a big reinforcer for something will work even if it is negotiated with the subject (e.g., gold stars for completing homework for school adding up to a new video game will work with some kids, or you might reinforce yourself with a special coffee, a dinner out, or a new shirt if you do a week or a month of Diary Cards 6 out of 7 days).

Presenting the Week 3 Assignment

1. Hopefully, clients will read Chapter 1 ("Reinforcement") of *Don't Shoot the Dog*. To encourage this, you might want to do a behavioral assessment of reading skills and motivation of the clients, and troubleshoot how those for whom reading is a challenge can use their skills to do this optional homework. Some clients may be more likely to listen to the "Hidden Brain" podcast on clicker training (Schmidt et al., 2018) than read the chapter.
2. The Week 3 Assignment: Practicing Reinforcement (pp. 38–41) provides an opportunity for clients to practice on their own what you practiced in class. Questions 2–6 are thought exercises. The clients work through the ideas for something they want someone else to change and something they personally want to change. Then they decide which one they want to attempt and try it. As always, we end the exercise with observations about the experience (p. 41).
3. Orient the client to hanging loose with this assignment—just explore it and experiment. You can't learn all of the behavioral therapy principles in a week. As highlighted in the "General Notes" for this module, if this is something that is important to what the client is working on in DBT Next Steps, their individual therapist can pick up on these skills and incorporate them more directly in individual therapy.

4. Use the skills from weeks 1 and 2 to approach this with high achievement or being average, rather than from a perfectionist mindset. The goal is to get the feel of it and illustrate the reading to improve class discussion, rather than to really change the other person. For example, if positive reinforcement of a roommate doing dishes didn't lead to many dishes being washed this week, the high achiever might reflect that "this will take some time, so let's see how it goes next week" versus the perfectionist who may think, "I failed at doing positive reinforcement."
5. Highlight that they should start the assignment (addressing Questions 2–4) with an example about someone else and then do Questions 5–7 about themself. It is easier to understand reinforcing someone else (note that they can choose a pet).
6. Encourage them to use positive, not negative, reinforcement to start out with. This first assignment should be about trying to positively reinforce someone else's behavior—it is easier and will result in the least resistance.

Reviewing the Week 3 Assignment

1. The challenge for the group leader is to find a synthesis of clarity and precision about the concepts (since practice with confusing or incorrect feedback is not helpful) and reinforce effort, creativity, willingness, and flexibility. If you go too far into the weeds of mistakes, you will punish the clients' efforts. On the other hand, clients generally make a lot of mistakes here, and you don't want to let them think they are correct. Orienting to this issue ahead of time, validation, reinforcement of adaptive behavior, and a light touch are needed. Modeling rather than dragging the behavior out of them can help, and it is important to reinforce effort.
2. If it doesn't appear that reinforcement occurred or the wrong behavior was reinforced, highlight that doing this is not so easy, yet hopefully with corrections it will make more sense. For those who are taking DBT Next Steps for a year, they will come back to this assignment in 6 months and give it another go. If their practice example seems relevant to their life, encourage them to follow up with their therapist because it may be worth revising and trying again.

Week 4: Untraining or Making It Stop!

Key Points for Teaching

1. This week is a switch from increasing behaviors to decreasing them—providing an overview of the ways in which reinforcement can be used to stop problem behaviors. There really is not enough time for clients to become competent with these ideas so it is important to orient them to the following: (a) This is just something you want them to have a general idea of and they can pursue more with their individual therapist if they want to, and (b) it would be ideal if they read Chapter 3 ("Stimulus Control") of *Don't Shoot the Dog* in addition to Chapter 4 ("Untraining") if they are interested in learning more.
2. The Week 4: Untraining or Making It Stop! handout (p. 42) describes the behavioral strategies of untraining as "Good Fairies" and "Bad Fairies" (see Chapter 4, "Untraining," of

Don't Shoot the Dog). One key concept is to get clients committed to the idea that "Good Fairy" options are out there and are the most effective. The other key concept is for clients to understand what isn't effective about the "Bad Fairies" but when they are still useful.

3. The exercise, as outlined in the teaching handout, is to work through two (preferably quite different) problem behaviors that the group identifies. The point is to have different answers to the eight methods of untraining and to see that for different types of problem behavior, different methods appear more likely to work.
4. The eight methods of untraining are described in detail in *Don't Shoot the Dog*, with Methods 1–4 being "Bad Fairies" and Methods 5–8 being "Good Fairies." While key points are highlighted below, it is expected that group leaders will have studied this chapter and will be competent in this area prior to teaching it.
5. Key teaching points for the "Bad Fairy" Methods 1–4 are:
   a. *Method 1:* Shoot the Dog—Eliminate the Problem or the Situation
      i. This method removes the subject's access to the behavior—they can't do it so the problem is solved. For example, if someone is caught breaking into someone's house and is put in jail, they can no longer break into a house. Or if you get divorced, your spouse can't bother you about whether you put the cap on the toothpaste.
      ii. The only time this method should be employed is when the subject's behavior is too major to endure and unlikely to be modified.
   b. *Method 2:* Punishment
      i. Doesn't work because subject learns nothing about how to change the behavior you want them to alter (they might be motivated to suppress whatever they were doing, although they don't learn what would be a better alternative, so they tend to freeze and do little at all, or feel cornered and fight).
      ii. "Trainer" learns to use punishment because it is reinforcing to the trainer, not to the subject. For instance, punishment can provide revenge when you feel wronged, demonstrates dominance, and if behavior is suppressed, there is relief for the trainer.
      iii. If punishment doesn't work, there can be no end to the escalation of the punishment, resulting in outcomes of fear, hatred, and evasiveness.
      iv. Guilt and shame are often used (consciously or unconsciously) by clients as a way to punish themselves for behaviors they don't like. However, as with any other punishment, the guilt and shame generally won't work because they come too late (i.e., after the clients have gotten the immediate relief or other immediate positive reinforcement for that behavior).
      v. The only time when punishment is likely to work is when behavior is new and caught early and when punishment is novel to the subject.
   c. *Method 3:* Negative Reinforcement
      i. In negative reinforcement, something the subject doesn't like can be "turned off" by the subject by doing a desired behavior. The classic example is nagging, which stops when the subject does the desired behavior (e.g., completes their homework, takes out the trash). Internally, relief is an important reinforcer to DBT clients—that is, a

negative emotion (fear, anxiety, anger, shame) goes down when they do a behavior (e.g., cutting, procrastinating looking for job postings).

- ii. Overuse of negative reinforcement does not lead to the hatred, fear, and evasiveness of punishment, although it can be associated with timidity, doubt, and anxiety in the subject unless balanced with a lot of positive reinforcement.
- iii. To reduce resistance, the subject needs to see the aversive and stopping the aversive as a consequence of their own behavior and not arbitrary, like punishment. Be sure to stop the aversive immediately when there is even slight improvement in the subject's behavior.
- iv. Negative reinforcement won't work with babies of all species since they will just get scared.
- v. It is ideal for deliberately willful behavior. In this case, the subject won't resent the negative reinforcement because they know their behavior is a problem (e.g., messaging a potential partner who isn't answering over and over until they respond).

d. *Method 4:* Extinction

- i. Extinction means stopping a reinforcer that has previously been trained with a behavior and now you want the behavior to stop. A cat is reinforced for crying at your bedroom door or sitting on your head because you get up and feed them. If you want to stop them from doing this, you need to extinguish the behavior—that means you have to stop reinforcing them by feeding them after behaviors you don't like. Maybe you start feeding them at the same time every day regardless of whether they cry or sit on your head.
- ii. Ignoring is a notable social action and may be more punishing or reinforcing than extinguishing. It is important to find a way to ignore the behavior (extinguishing) without ignoring the person (reinforcing or punishing).
- iii. Verbal behaviors such as whining, quarreling, and teasing tend to respond well to extinction. For example, if you ignore your young daughter's whining while continuing to provide for her basic needs (without giving her more attention when she's whining), the whining will extinguish for lack of reinforcement.
- iv. It is important to remember that when a previously reinforced behavior is no longer reinforced, extinction will occur, but often not until after an extinction burst (e.g., your daughter's whining will increase or turn into a tantrum before extinguishing for lack of reinforcement). The best response is to apply one of the "Good Fairy" strategies for the behavior you want instead, so that as they are deprived of reinforcement for the behavior you are extinguishing, they are simultaneously reinforced for something else (e.g., give a lot of attention and your focus to all nonwhining behaviors; see Method 7).

6. Key teaching points for the "Good Fairy" Methods 5–8 are:

a. *Method 5:* Train an Incompatible Behavior

- i. It is very hard to not do something or to avoid doing something. It is much easier to do something specific that is incompatible with the behavior you want to change.
- ii. To get a dog not to bark at the door, you can train it to sit quietly on a rug across the

room when the doorbell rings. Instead of reinforcing your mother for "not yelling," it may be easier to consistently reinforce her for "speaking softly." It is easier to get through a difficult time of day when you typically smoke by reinforcing yourself for doing something incompatible at that time (e.g., running, swimming), rather than trying to "not smoke during this time."

b. *Method 6:* Putting the Behavior On Cue
    i. This builds on natural law that when a subject practices doing *X* only after a *Y* cue, then *X* extinguishes when a *Y* cue is no longer presented. For example, if a dog is reinforced for asking to go out only when there is a towel on the door handle, then the dog will stop asking to go out whenever the towel is off the door handle (unless the dog really has to pee, in which case Method 8 applies).
    ii. The key to this method is to reinforce *X only* with a *Y* cue, and never otherwise. In this example, you'd have to put the towel on the door handle often enough that the dog has plenty of opportunities to go out with the towel, so you never have to respond to the dog asking to go out when the towel isn't there.
c. *Method 7:* Shape the Absence of the Behavior
    i. This method is much less complex than others and is a really useful strategy. It involves reinforcing any behavior other than the one that is undesirable. You therefore don't need to decide on a specific alternative behavior to increase or face the further complication of that behavior not occurring.
    ii. For example, if you decide that you are turning off your computer screens after 8 P.M. in your household, then you would reinforce any activity that doesn't involve a screen. That may mean reinforcing an extra snack, a walk you don't feel like taking, and so forth.
d. *Method 8:* Change the Motivation
    i. The key is that untraining just won't work unless you make an accurate assessment of what the motivation is for the subject's behavior. If you get it wrong, this method won't work at all.
    ii. Once you've determined the correct motivation, you have to decide if you can really eliminate the underlying cause or not. If not, then this is the wrong method for that particular situation.
    iii. If you do know the cause and it makes good sense to change the motivation, then this is exactly the way to solve the problem and will almost always work. For example, if you are in a carpool where people are being particularly grouchy or complaining and you believe this is because they are hungry, you could bring snacks to share. The general atmosphere might improve.

Presenting the Week 4 Assignment

1. Encourage reading Chapter 4 ("Untraining a Behavior") in *Don't Shoot the Dog.* Ideally, clients will read Chapter 3 ("Stimulus Control") as well.
2. The Week 4 Assignment: Untraining Behavior (pp. 44–45) is another thought exercise. The goal is to pick a behavior to untrain and apply the methods to that behavior.

3. Certain methods will be a real stretch for some behaviors. Orient the client to that fact if it wasn't already illustrated in the in-class example. Encourage creativity and being a little silly to make something fit. It is more important to understand the idea than to come up with something that one would actually do.
4. There isn't an expectation that clients go out and practice using any of the methods suggested, although you can encourage them to experiment and try something if they want to.
5. If clients try untraining a behavior that they previously reinforced, it is important to remind them there may be an extinction burst and not to give up.
6. Highlight for clients that it is time to complete a Self-Assessment of DBT Next Steps Recovery Goals (pp. 46–49). They should complete the handout and give it to their therapist, or bring it to group next week and the group leaders will pass on the completed form to the individual therapist. Remind clients that the goal is to take stock of their progress in DBT Next Steps and to be sure that their individual therapy is on track.

Reviewing the Week 4 Assignment

1. As this was a thought exercise, your goal is to be sure that the clients correctly identified an example for each of the methods that:
   a. is actually an example of that method
   b. actually fits the problem behavior they are trying to untrain
2. The goal is not that clients can go out and practice a specific untraining behavior based on this limited teaching, but to help them see that behavior in themselves and others follows predictable patterns. If they don't change how they respond to their own and others' behavior, then they will have to live with a lot of behaviors they don't like.
3. As with the previous week's homework, you are looking for a synthesis of clarity and precision in your teaching of the material, with reinforcement of adaptive behavior. The strategies described for reviewing the Week 3 Assignment apply here.
4. If a client actually tries the untraining behavior, ask for observations and reinforce courage and willingness as well as any creativity, flexibility, and the like.

CHAPTER 16

Module: Establishing and Re-Evaluating Relationships

General Notes

1. The majority of clients in DBT Next Steps do not have a social network and social support that are working well for them. They often have friends and family in their lives who don't promote their happiness and success, and are frequently without friends and family who do. This is consequently an important element of many client's ambitions. It is also a common goal on the Check-In: to find friends and a significant other/partner (as is normative for others their age).
2. The clients' life circumstances are generally changing in SDBT and DBT Next Steps, and their social networks need to change with them. These are also important skills over time as life circumstances will continue to change and clients may need to rebuild social networks more than once.
3. Many DBT Next Steps clients come to treatment with very narrow social experiences and may have avoided social situations after a history of failed relationships or fear of danger or humiliation. Social phobia is common. At the same time, a life worth living includes at least a few strong relationships.
4. Social connectedness is one of the most established protective factors against suicide. It is key that a client have people in their life who will reach out to them when they don't show up or stop calling; that they be an insider, not an outsider.
5. Many clients will say that they are loners and don't want a lot of friends. That is absolutely fine, and they should be encouraged to follow their Wise Mind. However, it is important

to distinguish between genuinely not wanting a lot of relationships in your Wise Mind and being unable to find, create, or keep them. The clients should be reminded that this is a skills-training module, and the skill is to find, create, and keep a social network. They should practice all the strategies and make steadfast efforts to do all the assignments regardless of whether or not this is what they want in their life in general. If they become competent in the skills and then choose not to use them after DBT Next Steps, this is their Wise Mind decision to make. However, during DBT Next Steps, we will ask them to be willing to learn and practice, so they have these interpersonal skills in their repertoire.

6. Co-leaders and individual therapists have to be sure that they themselves do not have hopeless thoughts or doubts about their clients' ability to achieve normative relationships. These doubts will quickly be transmitted to the clients who are vigilantly on the alert for this kind of feedback. In addition, therapists should be sure they aren't falling into a pattern of assuming that clients on psychiatric disability are unlikely to get married, have children, play a leadership role in their community, or be a trusted friend. Therapists should practice observing and describing the people they see around them in their own lives who fulfill these roles. It will quickly become evident that achieving these relationships is not rocket science and is certainly attainable by most DBT Next Steps clients.
7. Therapists who have hopeless thoughts should use the DBT consultation team to challenge and re-moralize them. This is an important function of the consultation team.

Week 1: Developing Accurate and Ideal Maps of My Community

Key Points for Teaching

1. This week's goal is to help clients accurately assess, that is, observe and describe, their social community. As with many DBT modules, assessment is often the most effective way to start.
2. This task tends to elicit a lot of judgment, which then has to be blocked. To preempt this, leaders may want to start with a brief mindfulness exercise that involves practicing observing clearly and kindly without judgment. Alternatively, the leaders can be particularly vigilant to judgmental language in the Check-In and assignment reviews, helping clients remember to describe without judgment beforehand.
3. Note also that this task will often bring on negative emotions of sadness, regret, and disappointment. These are often valid emotions about the current state of their social network, and clients should be coached to be mindful of these emotions as they appear, rather than push them away. They are often justified and can be effective in motivating the client to make changes.
4. By contrast, if unjustified or ineffective emotions arise—intense shame, anger, or anxiety—the clients should be coached to practice effective opposite actions so they are able to master them both during class and when they work on this task for homework.
5. Start by orienting the clients to the goal of maximizing the quantity and quality of relation-

ships in their life and stress how this is a normative task that everyone has to do (with or without conscious thought).

a. Highlight the importance of the skill of establishing relationships because life can change, you may have to move, your community might change if you get married, and so forth. It is important to be able to reassess and restart at any time in your life.

b. Also highlight that people change and relationships change, grow, or die. Part of mindfully attending to relationships is deciding which to prioritize and which to let go of.

6. Present the concepts of community and active and effective membership on p. 53 (the Week 1: Developing Accurate and Ideal Maps of My Community handout).

7. Group leaders can share their own examples to model identifying people and organizations who can be in your community. Try getting clients to consider a fuller range of ways in which they are, or can be, connected, including various types of individuals on a smaller scale and types of organizations on a larger scale.

8. Prompt the group for ideas about why "absence causes expressions of interest or concern" is an indication of active and effective participation in your community. For instance, clients may discuss their experiences attending religious services at the same place for many years, but that no one seems to know who they are. They might feel connected to their religion or religious beliefs, but we wouldn't consider their role in that community as active and effective from the point of view of establishing and maintaining important relationships. Compare this to the client who prepares the food to be served after the service or is on one or more committees for upcoming events. They are not only connected to their house of worship but are also more likely to build meaningful relationships with other members of the community. The same can be said for 12-step meetings—you can come and sit in the back and leave afterward without talking to anyone or you can provide service to the community in setting up for coffee or cleaning up after the meeting, for instance. When you engage actively and effectively in the community and you don't show up, people will message you or ask if anything is wrong when they see you again. This means that you are an insider not an outsider, and that is critical. One of the benefits of playing on a sports team or hiking with a structured group is that you are going to be active and engaged through the activity itself, which increases the experience of connection and affiliation. And being the one to help with the equipment or provide transportation to the event can turbocharge your engagement in the community and lead to much stronger relationships.

9. Review the Community Mapping (p. 54) and Sample Community Map (p. 55) handouts.

a. Teach the class the five levels of intimacy or closeness:

i. "Close to your heart" refers to those people whom you can rely on, feel most attached to, and want to be the central people in your life.

ii. "Key people in your life" refers to those people who help you maintain your sense of connection to your community, provide support when you need it, and share common interests in regular, predictable relationships.

iii. "Friends (including family)" are those with whom you have fun, share ongoing or periodic activities or social events, and have some personal conversations, but not those you feel are key to your social network. Friends implies a relationship you choose where there is a genuine fit (e.g., of style, interests, sense of humor) and may include family, but not all family will be friends. Family can be anywhere on the map.

iv. "Acquaintances with whom you want positive interactions" refers to people you are connected to more because of your role (e.g., they are coworkers, your neighbor, your postal carrier, your brother-in-law, member of your church or gym), rather than by who they are as a person. Alternatively, it could be that you feel close to them as a person and for whatever reason you don't think they are someone it is effective to have as a friend (e.g., they are using drugs, are an ex-boyfriend or your boss). In this case, it is not due to lack of skill that they aren't closer to you, but rather a Wise Mind decision on your part to keep your distance.

v. "People you do not want in your life" is a category for people who exist in your community (past or present) whom you have decided you do not want to interact with—not even as casual, distant acquaintances. These are people where it is best to end the relationship.

b. Physical proximity, frequency of contact, and duration of the relationship are important aspects to consider when deciding at what level you want someone to be, but they do not define the levels. More important is the sense of personal closeness, love/like, and the function of the person in your life.

c. Have everyone try their hand at completing the Sample Community Map handout (p. 55) to determine their social community. Directions and tips are provided on p. 54—including the relevant DBT Next Steps Recovery Goals to help clients link this exercise with their overall treatment goals—and a completed example is included in Appendix 4 of the *DBT Next Steps Skills Handouts* volume.

10. As a group discussion, have everyone start their own sample map. Discuss the choices and answer questions to be sure everyone is getting the hang of it.

a. Have clients start their map by adding people in their existing social community.

b. Then ask them to practice deciding where to place people who are not already in their social community. This could be a specific person like "Corine" or a type of person like "a close friend" or "a wife," or a group like "running buddies," "master gardeners," "mom's group," or "my in-laws."

c. Some people have no one in the center of the map as there isn't anyone in their current network they want to be that close to them, and they will need to add new people at that level. Others who can't say no to people who are nice to them may have lots of people in the center three layers, but then realize that these aren't the people they truly want in their community. Such clients may need to push those people out to the friend or acquaintance level and bring in new people like "the love of my life," "a best friend," "a group of writers who support each other," or "children."

d. Be alert to and block judgment and self-invalidation. Call it out when you see it and get the person to fix it so the whole group gets the point. Highlight to the group how judgments often appear when one takes on a task like this. Their job is to fix or let the judgments go every time they pop up. If a client gets into a judgment binge and can't stop, they should put the task down, walk around, or otherwise shake themself loose, and come back to the task when they are able to be mindful. This exercise is not an opportunity to rehearse their life's failures, blame others, think hopeless and helpless thoughts, or condemn themself. It is an exercise in mindfulness—allowing emotions and thoughts to come and go mindfully while they find Wise Mind about something very important.

Presenting the Week 1 Assignment

1. Review the Week 1 Assignment: Complete Maps Now and Ideal graphics (p. 56). This is an observe-and-describe assignment. Prior to making changes to their social networks, we are asking clients to assess what their social network is like Now and what it would be in an Ideal Wise Mind world. The DBT Next Steps Skills Handouts volume contains a sample Community Map in Appendix 4, which clients can review before filling in the two community maps for this assignment.
2. Instructions are provided on the handout and refer to the Now map (p. 57) and Ideal map (p. 58). Emphasize that this task is both to create accurate community maps (of current reality and of their ideal preferences) and a mindfulness exercise of observing, describing, and finding Wise Mind about an emotionally laden topic.
3. Encourage those who have been expressing distress in class to practice Problem-Solving and Cope Ahead of Time skills by developing a plan to manage their emotions during the exercise and do imaginal practice before they start to complete the assignment. If they appear distressed enough that leaders are concerned they can't do it without becoming overwhelmed with shame, blame, or self-invalidation, encourage them to start the exercise in individual therapy. Try not to fragilize them—don't recommend this approach when they could do it alone using their skills.
4. Remind those who have been through the Perfectionism versus Reinforcement module to be a high achiever and not a perfectionist to get the best results.

Reviewing the Week 1 Assignment

1. Use Question 4 on p. 56 to guide the discussion.
2. Assignments can be reviewed one client at a time by putting the map on the board (or making a map you can edit on a shared screen for telehealth group). A blank map is filled in by the group leader for the whole group to view by having the client describe their map and asking them pertinent questions to place everyone in the best spot. (The clients can also be empowered to share the screen to show their map or go to the board and draw their map out while providing some commentary, if the skills leaders believe they are sufficiently prepared and understand the concepts well enough to do so. If not, the client's work will have to be corrected repeatedly, which may be punishing.) This approach works well if there is plenty of time and reinforces the time and effort of each client to do the task. It also offers the opportunity to help identify errors or misunderstandings carefully for each individual. However, time is often short, and it is also effective to have everyone discuss their now and ideal maps together as a group, answering Question 4; sharing their own experience of making the maps, what surprised them, what differed between the two maps, and so forth.

3. The goal here is to reinforce the client's adaptive behavior of mindfully observing and describing their social network with reasonable objectivity. Also reinforce dialectical descriptions—not just all problems or no problems. Many of the dilemmas they will run into with the maps and their social networks are normative, but not all clients will realize that. Validating that the problem is normal or common (Validation Level 5) and perhaps self-disclosing where the leader has experienced it (Validation Level 6) can be helpful.

Week 2: Diving Into New Relationships

Key Points for Teaching

1. The mission is to weave a path between the need for change (i.e., to drag out new behaviors, as we say in DBT) during each week of the module and accepting the reality that relationships don't develop or change quickly. You don't want the clients to rush things in a way that will decrease their success.
2. One piece of Diving Into New Relationships (see handout on pp. 59–60) is to recognize that there are things to do to build relationships that explicitly involve others (e.g., go to the same place regularly, go to a meet-up, chat with someone you like at work). There are also actions you can take to make yourself better "relationship material" that don't involve others (e.g., be hopeful rather than hopeless, use skills of observation and description effectively to choose relationships to pursue, cope ahead of time with potential barriers, get better at GIVE and other interpersonal skills). The client has to get out there and be where potential relationships are while also being the kind of person whom others would want to have a relationship with.
3. This means using Wise Mind and not doing the homework so diligently that they overdo it (e.g., messaging a friend too often, asking someone out too soon, sharing too much information at a new club activity) and alienate potential relationships. There are a number of strategies that clients can practice once they've done all they can to directly augment a friend relationship. For instance, if someone wants to be more involved in their church, they can go to church for all major services and sign up for one or two church-related groups. If they tried to go to church every single day and talk to everyone around them, though, this could be a demonstration of poor skills. Instead, on the days they don't have a new task to do, they could prepare by reading over church literature, planning or rehearsing how to avoid self-pitying thoughts, or going to another setting and practicing looking up and smiling (if looking down is a typical problem they exhibit when meeting people).
4. Group leaders disclosing their own exposure examples of approaching new relationships can go a long way here. Examples of approaching while simultaneously having urges to avoid new relationships can model for clients that it is possible to dive into new relationships while still experiencing emotions such as fear, shame, and the like. In other words, you can engage in social behavior (practice exposure) even if the action urges of your emotion tell you not to.
5. The Finding and Getting People to Like You skill from SDBT (Linehan, 2025a, 2025b) can come in handy when diving into new relationships. Rereading the content there on open groups versus closed groups can help clients as they approach new social environments.

6. Highlight that "Diving In" is deliberately chosen language to emphasize the need for participating nonjudgmentally, one-mindfully, and effectively. Putting only a third or a half of your attention out there while keeping the rest inside your head with negative thoughts (self-pity, hopeless thoughts, blame, "shoulds," etc.) will not yield relationships. Not only will you miss cues and appear odd or distracted to others, but you are also sending out negative nonverbal messages that will push others away.
7. We've made up the term "psychotic optimism" that may be helpful here; that is, believing that things will work out despite all the evidence or your instinct that they won't. Some clients need "psychotic optimism" that they will find people whom they like and who like them. If you do not find this, practice reasonable as well as Wise Mind analysis of why not, so you can "fail well" and make "lemonade out of lemons." Figure out where the problem lies by observing and describing with a positive problem-solving stance and make relevant changes so your future attempts will be more successful.
8. Most initial bids for relationships don't work out. It really is like fishing; while there are a lot of fish out there, you still have to cast your line many times before you catch the right fish.
9. Highlight how the "Strategies for Finding Satisfying Relationships" (p. 59) enumerated in the handout include approaches that both involve interactions with others and activities that have to be done on one's own to (a) be prepared or (b) improve how satisfying you are to be in a relationship with. In other words, emphasize the need for balance between getting out there and being ready. Putting yourself out there too much without any preparatory work on yourself won't result in success; neither will lots of preparation without getting out there.
10. Highlight for clients the balance between "Preparing for Finding Satisfying Relationships," "Strategies for Finding Satisfying Relationships," and "Strategies for Making Relationships Satisfying" (pp. 59–60). Again, modeling by the group leader can help.

Presenting the Week 2 Assignment

1. Over the next 7 days, the Week 2 Assignment: Do One Thing Every Day toward New Relationships (pp. 61–62) should reflect a balance between doing things that involve other people and doing things to improve your own "relationship quality" and optimism.
2. Clarify that clients are *not* expected to form a new relationship in 1 week. They are exploring a range of strategies to see what works and how. These are then strategies they can continue doing on their own or with their individual therapist.
3. The assignment uses the Check-In strategies of observing what is effective and what emotions they are experiencing. All the Check-In guidelines apply. The goal is to help clients observe their own process: What did they do versus how did they get themselves to do it? What are they experiencing?
4. Most clients' thoughts about how to find friends are overly simplistic (e.g., "make a friend," "meet people at parties"), so they have been unsuccessful in their attempts. The hope here is that by getting them to do a small thing every day and making the daily task manageable, they can both learn the skills that most people use to find new friends or relationships and sustain them over time.

5. Clients might set the bar too high by expecting that they have 1 week to find best friends. Group leaders can highlight the range of what diving into new relationships looks like, from practicing more GIVE skill with your barista to attending a meet-up event and participating fully.
6. Consider ways to weave this skill into the ambitions and Action Steps that the clients have already put forth. Clients may have chosen Action Steps that involve preparing for or finding satisfying relationships, or making relationships satisfying. If so, group leaders can use this assignment as a way of approaching these Action Steps. For example, one participant had chosen an Action Step of meeting one potential community partner for a social justice cause. This assignment then gave her a new way of approaching the initial contact so that it was less of a "cold call" and more about finding satisfying relationships with a shared social justice value. She was able to use the skills in this module to move her ambition forward.

Reviewing the Week 2 Assignment

1. When reviewing this assignment, rather than having one client list everything they did, it can be helpful to go around the room, with each person revealing one day's strategy/effective/emotion and then moving on to the next group member for as long as you have time.
2. The leaders' goals are to:
   a. Clearly and precisely reinforce adaptive behavior, especially keeping steps small, persistence, being daring, overcoming negative/hopeless thoughts, being creative, being willing, and so on.
   b. Reinforce not only that someone met someone, but also the practice of daily skills.
   c. Highlight the common types of effective strategies that clients identify. These can be listed on the board as the clients generate them, with a checkmark next to any that are used more than once. This can help the clients recognize the most effective strategies.
   d. Highlight the emotions they experienced—normalize, validate, and reinforce all evidence of Wise Mind (rather than Emotion Mind) action.
   e. Highlight how effective strategies helped clients manage their emotions.
   f. Highlight and reinforce being effectively choosy about relationships as well as getting out there. Clients are often so relieved or grateful to have someone respond to them that they don't hold to their Wise Mind values and quality standards for the other person's personality or behavior.

Week 3: Re-Establishing Existing Relationships

Key Points for Teaching

1. This week, the focus is on how to decide what past fragile, avoided, lost, or damaged relationships to resurrect. This is primarily done by teaching mindful assessment: how to observe and describe the relationship nonjudgmentally, one-mindfully, and effectively.

2. It is difficult for most clients to do this. It requires a positive problem-solving stance and using Observe and Describe skills while consistently blocking assumptions and interpretations. It is also important to recognize the role of How skills.
   a. *Nonjudgmentally:* Lots of emotions are raised by past relationship mistakes and failures, which will generate a lot of judgments, shoulds, and blame toward self and others. However, the judgments will also generate emotions, so if they are not avoided, the client will be too emotional to do this task and the relationships will remain failed.
   b. *One-mindfully:* It is very difficult to assess one failed relationship without getting distracted by one's own failures in another area or other failed relationships. It is critical for the client to take one relationship at a time and not be distracted by other issues.
   c. *Effectively:* This is a prime place for right/wrong and fair/unfair to arise, and this will need to be blocked with some humor by the leaders. The clients will need to recall what their goal is: to be right or to figure out how to save or let go of a relationship.
3. Once the observing and describing are done, the goal is to practice using Wise Mind to choose what to do. The teaching ends with group practice for finding Wise Mind.
4. Remind the class that interpersonal skills have principles, but there is no "rulebook" or "recipe," so Reasonable Mind is not going to help that much. There is likely to be a lot of unhelpful emotion that arises, and running with that emotion will lead to behavior that we regret. Therefore, it is ultimately one's own personal Wise Mind that needs to make the call about each relationship.
5. Group leaders can magnify tension between two sides of the relationship: what clients liked about the person versus what they disliked. Try prompting for the other side and creating a synthesis if an example becomes polarized and reinforce group members for their dialectical thinking.
6. Ask clients to describe their body sensations as part of what they remember now about their reactions then (regarding previous interactions with a relationship they are considering re-establishing). The idea is to increase awareness of physical sensations as part of observing and describing emotions. If group members give vague responses, group leaders can try to prompt them for body sensations that are consistent with the emotions identified—for example, "You listed the emotion as shame, and thoughts like 'they don't care about me,' and I'm wondering if body sensation could have included a sinking feeling in your gut, or a heaviness in your chest. . . ."
7. Using the Week 3: Re-Establishing Existing Relationships handout on pp. 63–64, the first step is to help the group identify relationships that may need to be re-established and those that may not. These might be relationships that ended badly, have faded away, or where there is great ambivalence.
8. Talk about the idea of mindful assessment—using Observe and Describe skills with How skills to come to a meaningful Wise Mind decision they can act on consistently. Consider the idea of a dialectical assessment: What's being left out?
9. Use the Re-Establishing Existing Relationships handout to:
   a. Have each person work through a relationship in their life.

   b. Have a leader model with one of their lost relationships (using all DBT principles of self-disclosure as modeling), and/or
   c. Have the group work through one client's example.
10. Diligently focus on mindful Describe skills—blocking and reframing judgments, assumptions, and interpretations into facts or examples (e.g., by asking, "What makes you say that?" or "You may be right, but I'm wondering which facts led you to this conclusion?").
11. The handout offers useful prompts on what to describe about the relationship to be able to observe it effectively. What do they like? What do they dislike? How has the person supported or disappointed them?
12. The second section gets to the more intuitive and emotional side of the relationship and the impact of the relationship on the client.
   a. There are three private experiences to consider in the columns—emotions they experience, thoughts they had, and body sensations—as well as one public behavior, the actions they took.
   b. The handout asks about these experiences in three separate contexts with the other person:
      i. When they were feeling really connected/having a particularly good time.
      ii. When things were typical of how they are/were together—that is, not at a particularly wonderful moment, but the more typical or average times.
      iii. When things didn't go well.
   c. This 3 × 4 matrix provides a lot of information that can be used to make relationship conclusions. Some examples:
      i. The relationship could be full of extreme highs and lows, and though the highs are so great, the lows are so terrible that the person decides the relationship shouldn't be re-established.
      ii. While the lows are crushing and frustrating, the highs are so terrific and compatible with what makes the client happy that they decide to work on re-establishing the relationship with lots of problem solving or radical acceptance to manage the downtimes.
      iii. The person realizes that even during the lows, it was primarily their own thoughts and fears that got in the way, and if they can manage those, the relationship is worth it.
      iv. The person realizes that they never felt very positive emotions and body sensations with this person, so they let go of them.
13. Clients might reflect on their level of skill when they were in the relationship (pre-DBT) versus their level of skills now that they are in DBT Next Steps. Acknowledge that relationships can look quite differently once DBT skills are part of the equation, and not just interpersonal effectiveness. It's also the case that relationships can be stronger once Mindfulness skills are used to observe limits, emotions are more effectively regulated, and distress tolerance and radical acceptance are applied. Consider asking the group if they might show up in relationships differently as a result of DBT and get ideas about specifically how.

Presenting the Week 3 Assignment

1. The Week 3 Assignment: Accurate Assessment of Two Relationships (pp. 65–68) calls for practicing the strategies listed in the prior handout.
2. This assignment often brings up a lot of sadness and disappointment—primary emotions that make good sense given the circumstances. It is important for leaders to highlight the normality of this and demonstrate their compassion and empathy. If other clients do not naturally do so when it would socially be expected, they should be prompted to "read the room" and practice Validation skills from GIVE.
3. Clarify to the clients that this assignment is not about how a relationship would be re-established or whether that is possible. The goal here is to use Mindfulness skills to make a Wise Mind decision. Later, they can use their SDBT interpersonal skills if they decide to re-establish the relationship.
4. Clients will generally need coaching to regulate their emotions and practice a lot of distress tolerance, radical acceptance, and willingness to pull off this mindful assessment.

Reviewing the Week 3 Assignment

1. As usual, reinforcement of adaptive behaviors is key here—reinforce persistence in the face of emotion, creativity, willingness, emotion regulation strategies, radical acceptance, and so on.
2. If the client has had trouble or ended up writing down assumptions, interpretations, or judgments, the client should be prompted to turn them into descriptions.
   a. One exercise you can do here is to have everyone practice asking, together, "What makes you say that?" as a prompt for a description, rather than a judgment/assumption/interpretation.
   b. You can have everyone practice this before you start the review of the assignment, and then whenever anyone notices someone else making a judgment/assumption/interpretation, they can ask, "What makes you say that?" This question normalizes shifting from judgment to description. There is a commonly practiced DBT mindfulness exercise, "Shoe Mindfulness," that illustrates this (McCann, n.d.).
3. Try and work through at least one of each client's relationships. Ask at the end what their Wise Mind decision was. Validate what is valid about that decision, but avoid validating what does not appear to be valid. This is important modeling. Generally, this isn't difficult to do and often their process and decisions are quite moving.

Week 4: Variations on GIVE: Casual Conversation and Creating Distance

Key Points for Teaching

1. These skills present a range of options for intensity to consider in relationships and can often come in handy with people who are acquaintances or whom the client doesn't know

very well. The skills covered in this session involve a casual and toned-down use of GIVE for social gatherings, and the STOP skill to avoid and create distance from unwanted interactions.

2. The "Being Casual" section of the Week 4 handout (p. 69) describes the variations on GIVE and related strategies. This is a big change from week 3, which is about important and often emotionally laden relationships. Instead, the focus of week 4 is the "Acquaintances with whom you want positive interactions" from the Community Map. We aren't worried about forming or reforming relationships. We are concerned with a one-off situation like eating donuts after a church service; attending a cocktail party; going to a ball game, bar, party, break room; the social time that occurs after yoga class; and so forth. Situations where the clients are practicing being part of a community without a focus on any particular relationship.
3. For the "Too much information!" section (item 4), group leaders can use examples of striking the right balance of disclosure. One approach might be matching the other person in what they disclose and then adding slightly more information.
4. Group leaders can prompt the group for examples they have observed about "keeping it light" (item 5) and the "subtle shift" (item 6). Discuss ways in which people have mastered these strategies and the effect that has had on others. In other words, the clients should think about really socially skilled people they know and how those people might move the conversation on or end it in a casual manner.
5. Identify factors that get in the way of this type of interpersonal effectiveness: Is there unjustified guilt that comes with the idea of exiting the conversation, and if so, what are the skills from SDBT that are helpful to reduce unjustified guilt? Other factors could be lack of social skills in this arena or indecision about whether to stay or go.
6. The Finding and Getting People to Like You and Options for Intensity skills from SDBT (Linehan, 2025a, 2025b) can come in handy when doing a "toned-down" GIVE for casual conversations. Rereading the content about working on conversational skills and on open groups versus closed groups can help clients as they practice casual conversation.
7. Next, move to the STOP skills (p. 70). The focus here is keeping someone who is pushing for more in the "Acquaintances with whom you want positive interactions" level, or keeping or moving someone into the "People you don't want in your life" level.
8. STOP is an acronym for the opposite of GIVE skills: Sharp not Gentle, Thoughtless not Validating, Offended instead of Easy Manner, and Preoccupied instead of Interested. (*Note:* This skill was named before the STOP skill was added to Distress Tolerance in the second edition of the SDBT skills manuals (Linehan, 2025a, 2025b) and is a totally different skill.)
9. The STOP skill is used when the goal is to build distance from the other person and to get distance quickly. There is an art to avoiding interpersonal situations, and these are all ideas of things to do to get distance. Note that it can be about obtaining distance in the moment, even if you want to keep the relationship in the long run, and it can be used to get distance when keeping the relationship is not important.
10. Group leaders can bring up the idea that verbal communication should fit with nonverbal communication to maximize the effectiveness of the STOP skill. For example, a conversation

can be prolonged if someone continues to make eye contact, even while they have disengaged body posture, aren't talking to the other person, or appear preoccupied.

11. Clients can get quite anxious about using STOP skills if they believe they should be nice to everyone. Challenge this Interpersonal Myth as you would in SDBT. Help clients Check the Facts on how much they are really hurting the person by doing the STOP skill and what the relative hurt is to encourage them now, only to reject them later. Encourage them to find Wise Mind here and not to be mean or cruel in their enactment of STOP. That isn't necessary.
12. Practicing STOP skills during group is highly recommended (and usually hilarious). Have clients think of someone they would like to back off from (a panhandler at a bus stop, someone trying to pick them up at a party, mother butting into their private life on a phone call, sexual innuendo or harassment at work). Role-play in group. The group can coach during or observe afterward any GIVE skills that slipped in. Have the person try it again with less GIVE and more STOP, and see if the other person backs off more quickly. Reinforce the synthesis of kindness and firm use of STOP.
13. For clients who have been through the Perfectionism versus Reinforcement module, consider how inadvertently adding a validating statement or appearing interested with eye contact might be intermittently reinforcing the other person's behavior. If they are trying to block the behaviors with the STOP skill, consistency is important from a reinforcement standpoint.

Presenting the Week 4 Assignment

1. Go to the Week 4 Assignment: Casual Conversation and Creating Distance (pp. 71–73). The first part of the handout is a thinking practice: to help clients reflect on the recommended strategies. Then they will need to find at least three situations where they can practice all six strategies. As usual, the assignment ends with a request for observations.
2. Next, the clients practice STOP skills (p. 73). Again, the first step is for clients to put the skill into their own words. Then they practice it twice in separate situations.
3. Some clients spend so much time in socially uncomfortable or problematic situations they have no shortage of STOP opportunities. Often, however, one or both of these situations will need to be manufactured or planned ahead for clients who don't generally have occasion to use STOP twice in one week. For instance, a client might be encouraged to take a bus where they know that people will be more intrusive or a concert where someone is likely to encroach a bit too much on their personal space or a family gathering where an aunt is likely to ask too many nosy questions. (In the latter case, the client can alternate STOP when their aunt first becomes overly nosy with GIVE for the rest of the exchange so as to maintain the relationship.)
4. Even though STOP is designed to get distance from the other person and to obtain that distance quickly, clients may feel overwhelmed thinking they need to set out and reject people as part of the assignment. Highlight the range of what it looks like to use this skill. For example, STOP can be used in response to interpersonal behaviors where relationship effectiveness is a priority. That is, in situations where the relationship is important to

maintain, but the other person is engaging in behaviors that are challenging and/or offensive and it's important to get distance in the moment. One might practice STOP with a relative who is talking about politics at the dinner table in a dismissive or offensive manner, for example, and then move in with other skills to increase the connection at another moment when the behavior is not present. Challenge the ideas that might come up suggesting that to invest fully in a relationship is to be on board with ALL of the other person's actions ALL of the time.

5. The idea of the Week 4 Assignment is to extend clients' repertoire of responses across the Community Map.

Reviewing the Week 4 Assignment

1. Start the review of both the casual conversation and STOP skills with a discussion of the concepts. Compare how people describe the skills and where they are useful. Reinforce the range of relevant situations clients suggest as long as they make sense. If someone appears to be using the concepts incorrectly, either correct their understanding or highlight the valid parts.
2. Some situations will cause debate, depending, for instance, on how introverted or extroverted a client is. Highlight dialectics, but validate only the valid.
3. As always, reinforce practice, particularly the client throwing themself into being persistent and creative.
4. As relevant to client descriptions of their assignments, highlight for the class how over the course of this module clients have extended the range of their skills in social situations and relationships.
5. Reinforce increasing nuance in clients' observations and actions toward others and themselves.

CHAPTER 17

Module: Time Management Skills

General Notes

1. This module is directly tied to the Self-Sufficiency Recovery Goals, which will facilitate many other Recovery Goals.
2. Many concepts in this module, particularly the time map, are inspired by Julie Morgenstern's *Time Management from the Inside Out* (2004). Group leaders would benefit from reading this book ahead of teaching this module. However, over the years this module has become considerably more flexible than Morgenstern's ideas, which require considerable time, effort, and commitment to implement. We have found that our more flexible model has helped clients to understand and commit to the key principles of time management without getting hung up on the specific process Morgenstern recommends.
3. It is critical that group leaders have gone through the process of making ideal and current time maps for themselves before teaching this module. You can't explain something as unfamiliar as a time map if you have never tried it. Follow the guidance in this module, and you can also read or watch Morgenstern's (n.d.) other materials for more information. Over the years, her website has offered different versions of the time map you can try if you want to do it her way. Do not try and do a time map in one sitting just before you teach this module. It will be extremely frustrating and ineffective. Practice doing several, stopping for a while, coming back to them, and so on. This is a Wise Mind exercise, which is extremely Reasonable Mind while you are doing it, and you need to step away and let Emotion Mind stew on your plan for a little while to find Wise Mind. When you come back to it, you repeat this Reasonable Mind work and Emotion Mind "cooking," until you have that deep Wise Mind sense that you are there because when you come back to it there is not much you want to change (as we do to find Wise Mind about other things). This is how you want to coach the clients to do it, too.

4. We are not expecting our clients to create and adhere to a time map as we would expect them to practice Mindfulness or Opposite Action skills—all the way. Some people will really embrace the time map, but most clients will go through this process, learn a lot about time and how they spend it, and never use a time map outside of group homework.
5. Many clients struggle with this module. They aren't used to the idea of being so busy they have to make hard choices on how to spend their time, or they may be generally willful about this. We have found if the clients are doing DBT Next Steps for 1 year and will go through these skills twice within that time, it is best to take it easier the first time through. Clients will get into the module more the second time around.
6. Individual therapists should be aware of when this module is being taught, so they can build on it or modulate the demands of it, depending on their Recovery Goal targets and where the client is in the course of treatment.
7. This module provides grids for both the activity log and time maps in case clients prefer to work that way, but electronic tools such as Google or Outlook calendars or time-tracking apps, like Daylio, are often much easier to use than these grids. The grids can be ignored if not needed.

Week 1: Assessment of Time versus Values and Ambitions

Key Points for Teaching

1. The handouts for this lesson (pp. 77–79) build on time management from the inside-out concept of your time being equivalent to a closet—there is only so much space, but we could organize it better and get more inside. Time is equally fixed but less tangible. People generally know this in their Reasonable Mind, but day to day they act as if time is expandable. This exercise is designed to help clients experience their week as a fixed amount of time.
2. The time bar on p. 77 of the week 1 handout shows a week's worth of time with 112 hours that are waking and 56 hours that are sleeping. The right side of the page lists common categories of how people's time is spent.
3. We generally start by walking clients through the ideas and letting them start guessing at numbers in the blanks on the right side of the page. This gets them oriented to the basic ideas.
4. We then take a look at the completed example on p. 78 of the week 1 handout, where the numbers have been used to divide up the 112 waking hours. This gives a more visual understanding of how time is spent.
5. Then we come fresh to the same task on p. 79, where everyone mindfully records their schedule of the best estimates. This iterative nature of new handouts encourages clients to start fresh, rather than get stuck on what they first decided. This task really needs to be done with a pencil or using an online calendar or multiple copies of the handouts, so the client can pause and take a fresh look. If they keep trying to make a single version of a time bar work and are faced with edits and cross outs that confuse matters, they'll get stuck.

Presenting the Week 1 Assignment

1. Orient the clients to the fact that this module has more time-consuming homework than most modules and do some troubleshooting about how clients will get it done. Now, turn to the Week 1 Assignment: Assessment of Time versus Values and Ambitions.
2. The first task for the week (Question 1, p. 80) is to once again take a fresh look at the time bar for another try at their time estimates. They will have time during the week to complete some of the calculations they don't have time for in group and get a chance to observe themselves moving through the week and see what they actually do.
3. The second task (Question 2, p. 81) tracks how they spend their time over the course of the week. This information makes time maps a much better approach than when the client just comes up with subjective estimates of where their time goes.
4. We encourage the use of electronic tools to track time. This is something that many professions that bill by the hour need done, so there are a range of simple to complex time trackers available for smartphones. If this is not a fit for a client, a simple grid Activity Log is provided as part of the assignment handout for clients to use (pp. 83–84), or they can create their own. Clinicians familiar with behavioral activation will recognize this as the activity portion of a Mood and Activity Log. (Adding mood actually makes this process more effective, so clinicians can decide on that choice on a case-by-case basis; however, we have found that this week generates a lot of homework, so we generally simplify the task to only include activity.)
5. The third task (Question 3, p. 81) asks clients to explicitly bring their ambition and values into the picture for generating a time map (which is the task for week 2). This first week, we ask them to restate their ambitions and then add values (which is now part of SDBT, so we refer to that handout).
6. The final task of the week (Question 4, p. 82) requires clients to make observations of the results of the first three tasks, which will, in turn, help them make a plan for their time going forward.

Reviewing the Week 1 Assignment

1. The first task of the group leaders in reviewing this homework is contingency management to be sure clients are doing all the assignments in this module. It is more work than most modules so, having oriented last week, now is the time to hold people accountable, reinforce hard work, and conduct missing-links analyses where assignments are undone or incompletely done.
2. The main focus of the review of assignments here in addition to contingency management is:
   a. Ensuring that clients understand and have come up with an effective time-tracking strategy (Question 2). This will be done weekly throughout the module.
   b. Focus on Question 1 where they observe what changed about their time bar once they had time and space to think about it during the week, and Question 4 helping clients look across all three tasks and see what insights they can find.

Week 2: Developing an Ideal Time Map

Key Points for Teaching

1. Week 2 is built around the idea of a time map (see its description on p. 85 of the *DBT Next Steps Skills Handouts* volume). The time map is an ideal tool for DBT because it is very dialectical—balancing structured and unstructured activities, effort and ease, and things for others and things for yourself.
2. As DBT Next Steps clients shift from disability and dependency to meaningful employment, everything about time has to shift. Generally, we find DBT Next Steps clients are very happy to be working and/or in school. After about 5–6 weeks of this increased activity, they build the stamina for it. Sometimes they then overcorrect as they are encouraged to take more shifts or register for more classes and end up outside their limits (functionally self-invalidation). If they and their therapist can't anticipate this occurring and correct it, there is a risk of quitting. One way to avert this is to facilitate Wise Mind time management that considers all the things they may not be attending to, including household chores, commuting, downtime, leisure time, social relationships, and the like as well as their work and school activities, so they can see how much time they really have and "right-size" their job and school.
3. A time map is designed to give time some structure, like the dimensions of a closet. You can tell that your physical space has edges—a closet cannot be bigger than it is. You can fit more in the closet by organizing it more effectively, but there is a fixed limit. You can see the limit all the time as you go through the process of organizing it. When we think about time, we can't look at the edges of it like we can if we look into an empty closet. So, we get lost in trying to organize and fit the right amount of things into something we can't see all at once. A time map is designed to help us see the whole picture at the same time.
4. A time map is generally made around a week where the entire week is laid out and cut into blocks for all the different activities so you can see what fits and what doesn't. This is like putting shelves in a closet to separate spaces, or cutting out paper squares for furniture on graph paper to reorganize your living room, or using an app to design your garden. You decide how big each activity is (e.g., work, commuting time, grocery shopping, time to read a book, sleep), and you place them on the map and move them around until everything fits or you radically accept that somethings won't.
5. It is critical that group leaders understand the difference between a time map and a schedule, and then convey this to their clients. A schedule includes the specific activities and tasks you are scheduled to do—either because they are set (e.g., work hours) or tasks you know have to happen this week (e.g., get an oil change for your car). Schedules are tied to dates and thus not helpful for looking at the big picture. A time map is a general structure for time that is not at all tied to dates; it could represent any time and doesn't have any specific events listed on it. Specific events confuse the mapping process, like designing your living room for the whole year by putting a Christmas tree on the map—it will be an odd hole the rest of the year. Likewise, a time map is way too general (and often too full) to actually use as a schedule. Most people don't want their lives mapped out to this great a degree. The goal is to first see how everything fits and only then build your schedule. That way, your schedule is not dominated by specific events of the moment, but instead balanced by the big picture.

6. There are a range of time maps illustrated on Julie Morgenstern's website (www.juliemorgenstern.com); they also can be found by typing "time map morgenstern" into any search engine. Additionally, there's a sample ideal time map included in Appendix 5 of *DBT Next Steps Skills Handouts*. It is also fine if a client's time map is nothing more than a fully thought through time bar from week 1. If their time management is really straightforward, they can just keep the time bar handy as they build their weekly schedule and be sure they stay in balance with it. On the other hand, there are clients who have multiple demands on their time (e.g., work + school or complicated commuting + child care + a job) or who are more ambitious, and we don't want to fragilize them by not encouraging a more ambitious approach. It also helps people to recognize all the different categories that are in their life (or could be) during their ideal time map practice. Coach clients to radically accept their time-management needs effectively and without judgment, self-invalidation, or hopeless thoughts. Individual therapists can help here.
7. In week 2 (as shown on p. 86), we start with an ideal time map to assist the client to disengage from the day-to-day demands of their current life and see the big picture as it coincides with their values and ambitions. Group leaders will need to make a point of orienting clients to this and continually coaching them to see the forest, not the trees, for their initial view of the time map.
8. A time map is supposed to focus on one's values and ambitions first and accommodate the demands of life second. That is why we asked clients to remind themselves of their ambition and values as part of the Week 1 Assignment—so they have them in the front of their mind for this task.
9. Spend the teaching time for this week talking through the time map process, providing perspective and modeling as well as troubleshooting from your own experience of making a time map.
10. End the teaching by helping the group observe and anticipate worry thoughts, and troubleshoot both opposite action and check the facts strategies to counter them.

Presenting the Week 2 Assignment

1. The first part of the Week 2 Assignment (#1, p. 87) is for clients to continue with the Activity Log or time-tracking app from the Week 1 Assignment to keep self-monitoring their time. If they struggled with the Activity Log during the past week, do some troubleshooting and use commitment strategies.
2. The second task (#2, p. 87) is to make an ideal time map. As noted above, the format is entirely up to the client, and they should create whatever they think will be most effective. The key is the link it to their values and ambitions, while accommodating basics like grocery shopping, housecleaning, and commuting, plus things like self-care and downtime, which are critical to a balanced life. If clients would rather not use a standard grid and prefer to make a collage or picture to capture it, that's great, as long as they can see all of their time at once (i.e., they should not record a video).
3. As always, we end with observing and describing the process (#3–5, pp. 87–88).

Reviewing the Week 2 Assignment

1. If a client has not made a time map or tracked their time, assertively do a missing-links analysis and consider it as avoidance as you would in the Check-In. Highlight the dialectic of how important it is to engage with time management and how normative it is to avoid it. Suggest the client discuss this with their individual therapist if they aren't sure how to overcome the avoidance.
2. Review the clients' observations about their Activity Log/time tracking (#3, pp. 89–90).
3. Review each person's ideal time map (#4, p. 88). Ask how their values and ambitions are reflected in the map. Highlight where downtime and self-care are (or are not) on the map, and how they decided what was the effective amount of each to include and in what forms.
4. Reinforce smart ideas, creativity, flexibility, persistence, and willingness.
5. Review clients' observations about making the time map (#4, p. 88) and what worry thoughts interfered (#5, p. 88). Troubleshoot how to be effective with these issues going into the Week 3 and 4 Homework Assignments.

Week 3: Moving from an Ideal Time Map to a Trial Time Map

Key Points for Teaching

1. This week's practice involves moving from an ideal time map to something that clients can actually put into use. Have the clients put their ideal time map in front of them as you go through the questions on p. 93, which are self-explanatory.
2. Keep making the distinction between a time map and a schedule, so clients don't make the trial time map into a schedule. We still don't want specific events; we will do that part in week 4. The goal is to maintain a big picture map of time, just one that is more practical for the client's current situation.

Presenting the Week 3 Assignment

1. In the Week 3 Assignment (p. 95), continue the time-tracking task (#1) and make a trial time map (#2).
2. Sometimes, during the Week 2 Assignment, clients get stuck on a particular format for their time map that isn't working for them. Often, they will get new ideas from how others made their maps. Encourage them to change their format if they want to.
3. Once again, the assignment will conclude with observations that clients should make at the end of the week (#3–5, pp. 95–96).

Reviewing the Week 3 Assignment

1. As in previous weeks, if a client has not tracked their time (#1, p. 95) or made their time map (#2, p. 95), assertively do a missing-links analysis and consider it as avoidance as you would in the Check-In. Identify which emotions are interfering.

2. Review clients' observations in their Activity Log/time tracking (#3, p. 95) on what they noticed about their time this week.
3. Review each person's trial time map (#2, p. 95). If not clear, ask what the main changes were from the ideal time map. Be sure their values, ambitions, downtime, and self-care are still reflected in it. If not, troubleshoot how to restore them.
4. Reinforce radical acceptance, smart ideas, creativity, flexibility, persistence, and willingness.
5. Review clients' observations about creating the trial time map (#4, p. 96) and what strategies they used to effectively overcome any worry thoughts (#5, p. 96). Highlight that such effective ideas might be applied by others in the group.

Week 4: Moving from the Trial Time Map to Your Schedule

Key Points for Teaching

1. The teaching this week (see the handout on p. 101) focuses on standard time management strategies for effectively using a schedule. First, common time management guidelines for making a schedule are described, followed by some tips for being effective when scheduling tasks instead of appointments.
2. It is not expected that the schedule and time map will be identical. For example, even though someone would like to have a plan on Saturdays to hang out with friends and built this into their time map, this may have to be scheduled. Or maybe the client is behind on homework for school and will need to stay focused on that for a few more Saturdays before they will have time to hang out with their friends. Or perhaps they don't yet have friends to hang out with and the schedule needs to include activities to find friends, and maybe these activities don't happen to occur on a Saturday. At the same time, it is generally possible to bring more than half the time map into the schedule.
3. A principle from Julie Morganstern's (2004) book is that tasks need to be listed as appointments if enough time will be available to do them. So, you can't have your "closet" of time filled with work, appointments, and the like and then have a separate to-do list with tasks because there is no "place to put them" and thus no time to get them done. If you face the task of writing a résumé, sending holiday cards, planning a vacation, or getting the tires replaced on your car, these tasks have to fit somewhere, so your schedule has to include them as appointments.
4. The bulk of the teaching is providing effective information to clients on how to think about traditional time management now, after they have had time to think through their time map's big picture. The goal is to follow some or most of these strategies and bring the time map into creating a schedule, but it will take most of the teaching time to review the time management strategies.
5. Again, modeling from the group leaders about how they have effectively used these strategies, as well as how challenging they find them, is very helpful.

Presenting the Week 4 Assignment

1. As in previous weeks, the clients track time for 1 more week (#1, p. 103). Highlight that it will be interesting to compare and contrast this information with the newly revised schedule.
2. To close the loop, clients should make any final changes they want to their time map and keep a clean copy to try for a while (#2, p. 103. They may be happy with what they came up with in the Week 3 Assignment, in which case they will not need to change it again.
3. The main part of the Week 4 Assignment is to rebuild a schedule and to-do list using the time management principles and reflecting the principles of the time map (#3, p. 103). Remind clients of how the schedule and time map differ and to use the Revised Trial Time Map That Balances Feasibility with My Values and Ambition (pp. 107–108) as a structure, but adapt as appropriate to the specifics of the week. Encourage clients to work on their schedule soon so they can use it as much as possible during the week.
4. Use the schedule they came up with during the week and include guidelines discussed in class that are relevant to them (#4, p. 103).
5. Finally, there are a few observations to make at the end of the week (#5–7, p. 104).

Reviewing the Week 4 Assignment

1. If clients continue to not complete their assignments (#1–4, p. 103)—which happens more often in this module—identify missing links and emotions interfering and link these to their goals. Refer clients to their individual therapist if necessary.
2. Review the clients' observations on their Activity Log/time tracking versus schedule (#5, p. 104) with regard to what they noticed about their time this week.
3. Review each person's schedule (#3, p. 103). Discuss what parts of the time map made it into the schedule and what didn't. Be sure at least some of their values, ambitions, downtime, and self-care from the time map made it into their schedule. If not, troubleshoot how to fit them in.
4. Discuss how it went to follow their schedule and what guidelines or DBT skills they implemented to use their schedule effectively (#4, p. 103).
5. Reinforce radical acceptance, smart ideas, creativity, flexibility, persistence, and willingness.
6. Ask for observations (#5–7, p. 104).
7. Offer encouragement for continuing time management now that this module is over.

CHAPTER 18

Module: Managing Emotions Effectively

General Notes

1. Emotion regulation is core to SDBT, and DBT Next Steps presumes that the client knows and uses these skills regularly. The focus is the application of emotion regulation skills to the work, social, and self-management Recovery Goals to make them more achievable and to maximize the Emotional Proficiency Recovery Goals.
2. Week 2 of this module involves the client engaging with the individual therapist. As the therapist may be focused on other topics, it is helpful to alert the client that they should DEAR MAN their therapist for time to discuss the assignments in this module and/or orient the therapist that there are DBT Next Steps assignments to review.

Week 1: Assessment of Reducing Vulnerability Skills: What's Working and What's Not, and How to Change It

Key Points for Teaching

1. Re-orient clients to the idea of reducing emotional vulnerability and the critical need to maintain a low level of baseline emotion so that (a) one is not emotionally exhausted and (b) spikes of emotion caused by life circumstances start at a low enough point that they don't cross the skills tipping point.
2. This can be highlighted with the graph in Figure 18.1: Subjective Units of Distress Scale (SUDS; Foa et al., 2007; Wolpe, 1969, 1990). This graph should be drawn out for the clients on the board or shown on a shared screen for telehealth. Clearly, the top line is a worst-case scenario where the baseline SUDS never gets below 40; thus when it spikes, it goes

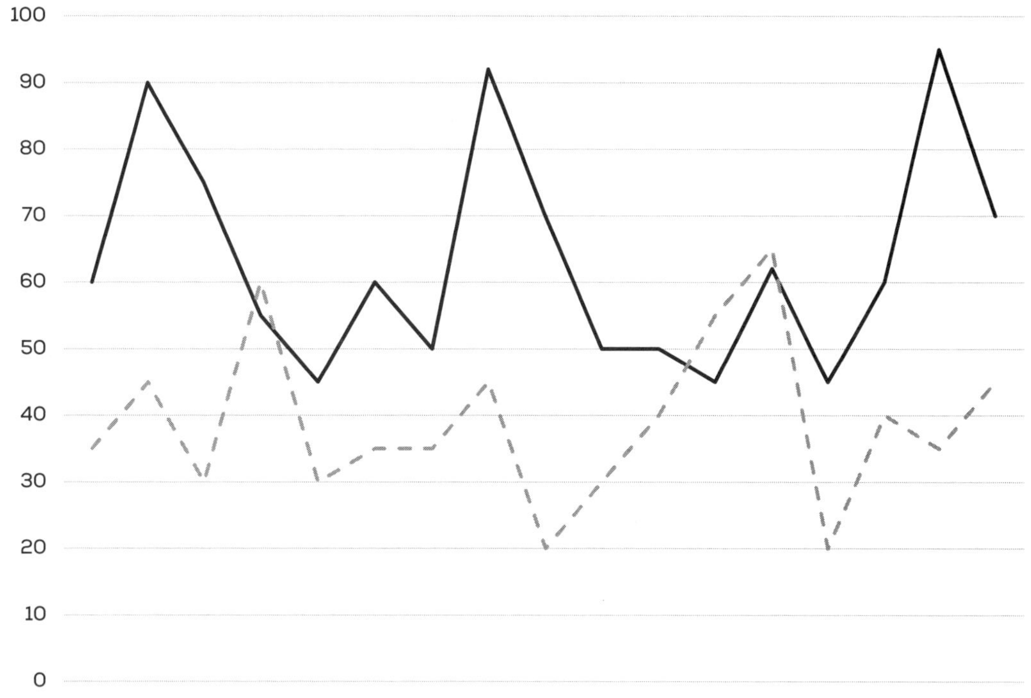

FIGURE 18.1. Subjective Units of Distress Scale (SUDS). Based on concepts from Foa et al. (2007) and Wolpe (1969, 1990).

so high (90–95 SUDS) that Emotion Mind action becomes increasingly likely. The lower line represents emotions in the presence of many Reducing Vulnerability skills where the average SUDS is more like 40 and the peaks never exceed 60–65. Essentially, the Reducing Vulnerability skills bring down the overall line.

3. The goal of Reducing Vulnerability is not to prevent spikes per se (although this may also happen) but to keep the baseline low enough that spikes are not a catastrophe.
4. It is important to normalize the importance of Reducing Vulnerability skills (i.e., provide your own examples of Emotion Mind behavior that was primarily caused by lack of Reducing Vulnerability skills). Also, normalize the difficulty of achieving and maintaining these skills, which is the bane of most individuals in the industrialized world.
5. Review the Week 1: Assessment of Reducing Vulnerability Skills: What's Working and What's Not, and How to Change It handout (pp. 111–112) in class. Highlight that the clients were already doing some of these skills pre-DBT, are no doubt practicing many of these skills, and have made gains since starting DBT. However, this assessment is designed to overview all these skills and help the client focus on where the best "bang for the buck" is likely to be in further strengthening these skills.
6. Another focus of this handout is to generalize the Check-In concepts to identify what is effective in getting these skills done and the large role of avoidance. Leaders should facilitate a discussion about troubleshooting: Consider how one client's effective strategies with one skill could help another client overcome their avoidance of another skill.

7. The exercise also teaches clients to observe their behavior nonjudgmentally and to do their own behavioral assessment. Be sure to go through several examples in class to be sure they understand the concepts and the handout directions.
8. Remind the clients that Cope Ahead is a combination of problem solving and imaginal practice (imaginal exposure). First, one identifies an upcoming situation that could cause emotion dysregulation and uses problem-solving skills to generate effective coping strategies for best- and worst-case scenarios. Second, one imagines the situation in the present tense and through one's own eyes. They imagine using the coping strategies effectively and also imagine things going wrong and coping effectively with that. This imaginal practice is repeated many times prior to the situation to maximize the likelihood that the skills will be used. This also serves as exposure to the cue. Many clients treat Cope Ahead as the Problem-Solving skill, which is useful but not as much about Reducing Vulnerability. The imaginal practice does that.
9. The next goal of this lesson is to give clients a model of how to systematically change health behaviors and other Reducing Vulnerability skills (pp. 113–114). Most people find this very difficult to change. The model we use is a variation of the Check-In as described in Chapter 14. The idea is to use behavioral theory to identify a feasible target, link to goals, use effective strategies to achieve the target, and avoid avoiding.
10. It may be useful for group leaders to reread the Check-In teaching points covered in Chapter 14 before teaching this module to be sure these concepts are fresh and easy to articulate. Orient the clients to the use of the Check-In steps here and that we are doing this because it is an established way to achieve a difficult goal or ambition.
11. The handout for this session (pp. 113–114) orients the clients to the difficulty of changing Reducing Vulnerability skills, particularly normalizing the difficulty, as in SDBT.
12. For this purpose, we use the word "goal" rather than "ambition" as we want something more circumscribed. The goal should be something that the client will experience as a real benefit of using the particular Reducing Vulnerability skill they selected (i.e., something more than being "good for them").
13. However, this works best if you start with a Reducing Vulnerability skill they will try (equivalent to the action step) first and match a goal to it, rather than picking a goal first. This is because they need to practice that skill rather than select any Action Step relevant to a goal, as is done in the Check-In.
14. Effective strategies and avoidance are identical to the Check-In. On the handout, they are stated in hypothetical terms ("What could I do?") in order to practice troubleshooting.
15. Work through an example in the group. Often, an excellent teaching example comes up in the self-assessment discussion and the skills leader can refer to that example. Alternatively, if you have a very quiet group or clients who have difficulty talking through a hypothetical example, the skills co-leader can offer to work through an example that is difficult (but not impossible) for them (i.e., acting as a coping model).
16. The mission in working through the example is to ensure that the clients see how each item from the Check-In is used to practice the Reducing Vulnerability skill with which they have difficulty.

Presenting the Week 1 Assignment

1. The first part of the Week 1 Assignment (p. 115) is to complete the self-assessment they started in class (pp. 111–112). Encourage them to review a draft with their individual therapist for any ideas that they might have missed.
2. Based on this assessment, the second part of the assignment is for the client to observe and describe their current use of Reducing Vulnerability skills through the week. Examples of what to track are described.
3. Coming from the time tracking in the time management module, this process of tracking something every week is familiar—but this time they only have to track Reducing Vulnerability skills, not all the other things they are doing.
4. *Note:* For many clients tracking their food intake is time- and energy-consuming or goes down an emotionally sensitive path that can distract from the overall mission of understanding Reducing Vulnerability. Therefore, clients are encouraged to note *when* they eat and not *what* they eat. (Individual therapists can have clients track what as well as when they eat if that is relevant to individual therapy targets.)
5. A Reducing Vulnerability Skill Tracking Calendar is provided (pp. 117–118) to assist clients in logging when they did each Reducing Vulnerability skill. Alternatively, many clients have now developed an effective calendar or planner system and would prefer to track these skills there, or they might like to use a self-monitoring smartphone app as they did for tracking time in the Time Management module.
6. The final part of the assignment is to pick a Reducing Vulnerability skill that the client finds challenging but would lead to a goal they would like to achieve. The assignment (pp. 115–116) then guides them through the Check-In process to increase their ability to practice that skill.

Reviewing the Week 1 Assignment

1. When clients review the self-assessment and week of tracking of their Reducing Vulnerability skills use, it can be helpful to do this with the group as a whole, rather than going person by person.
2. Ask the group as a whole, "Who learned something they didn't realize? Where did you see exactly what you expected to see? What surprised you? Which skills were you doing most? What skills did you find yourself avoiding?" After each question, pause for input from the clients. Generally, most clients will end up discussing the first two parts of the assignment.
3. If a client does not speak, skills leaders can prompt them by asking, for example, "Maria, what did you learn doing this assignment?" or something similar.
4. Skills leaders should reinforce new insights and hard work on this assignment and ask if anyone had trouble with part of it to provide additional guidance.
5. The best way to review the Check-In assignment is to go around the room, just as is done for the weekly Check-In because this is a very familiar format.

6. Key teaching points to highlight include:
   a. Benefit of problem definition—stating the skill precisely so you know when you are done.
   b. Linking to goals—when and where did remembering or visualizing the goal help complete the task.
   c. What are commonalities of the effective and avoidant behaviors that clients identified? It can be helpful to start a list of Effective Behaviors and Avoidant Behaviors as the clients report what happened when they did the assignment. Whenever something comes up a second time, put a check next to it. This highlights commonalities.
   d. Problem solving and troubleshooting avoidance; be sure that avoidance behavior is not treated as inevitable.
   e. Validating the normative difficulty of the task and how many other priorities can interfere or how emotions can talk clients into avoidance.
   f. For those who have done the Reinforcement module, highlight how there is often not an immediate reinforcement after doing the skill (except relief from guilt, shame, and/or anxiety) and that the lack of immediate positive reinforcement makes persistence difficult.
   g. Discuss effective strategies like public commitment, token economy, self-monitoring, doing it with a friend, and the like that may help here. Highlight how these are the same strategies used by, for instance, personal trainers or life coaches.

Week 2: Regulating Yourself When You Need It

Key Points for Teaching

1. As in Week 1, this session involves clients first doing an assessment of their problem areas (pp. 119–120). This is primarily because emotion dysregulation is such a core problem in DBT that it has been treated from many angles. Many areas of emotion dysregulation have been resolved prior to coming to DBT Next Steps or are resolved by the time the client gets to this module.
2. This assessment focuses on three core areas that are central to the Recovery Goals—work/school, social contexts, and self-management—and asks for an assessment of remaining problem areas in these contexts. This is important for the group to review, but is also very helpful in focusing the client and their individual therapist on the problem areas that still need attention.
3. The group should review the examples and add their own. Sometimes, it works to have the clients go around the room, with each one giving an example to get everyone involved. Other times, the skills leader will read through all the options and have the clients identify which apply to themselves or—if time is short—have the clients review the list themselves and identify the problems they have.
4. Validate and reinforce their progress in all the areas that no longer apply to them.

5. Challenge clients who see themselves as having problems in areas that aren't apparent to the group leaders, and try to find dialectical balance by being very specific about what the problem is and avoiding global thinking—for example:

   > "I'm not sure I get it, Joan. . . . You are describing obsessing and doing too much at work. But you focused on that in Check-In for a long time and moved on to other employment steps because you'd stopped doing it. Did you have a relapse we didn't know about? [Get feedback from the client.] OK. I get the problem—but it isn't obsessing or overdoing. I wouldn't check those problems, but you could add a problem: urges to overdo (which I don't act on) trigger dysregulation about other things."

   Precision is key, as the more precisely defined the problem, the more quickly and effectively the client will be able to use skills to resolve it.

6. The next step of this week's lesson is to plan ahead for problems that dysregulate the clients using an adaptation of the SDBT flowchart (Linehan, 2025a, 2025b) from Check the Facts to Opposite Action versus Problem Solving or Mindfulness of Current Emotion (pp. 120–121).

7. Situations are divided using the Check the Facts skill into two categories: situations where emotions are justified at this intensity and duration, and situations where they are not.

   a. Emotions that are effective at their current intensity and duration (e.g., "I'm embarrassed by my boss's criticism during a staff meeting") are addressed by problem solving the cue or practicing Mindfulness of Current Emotion. Problem Solving could mean changing the cue itself (e.g., asking the boss to give criticism in private) or, more often, changing the client's response to the cue (e.g., focusing on how everyone is criticized in meetings by their boss instead of their own criticism; blocking self-invalidating rumination or worry about the criticism; imagining the criticism being spoken in a chipmunk voice; focusing on observing which criticisms in meetings actually relate to job consequences rather than assuming this). Alternatively, it may not make sense to change the situation or their response to it, but instead to practice being mindful of their emotion as it is—focus on the feel of the emotion in their body (rather than their thoughts or the situation) and notice the sensations come, peak, and fade away.

   b. Emotions that are not effective at their current intensity and duration (e.g., "I'm humiliated by my boss's criticism during a staff meeting and my face is hot, my heart is pounding, and I have lost the thread of the conversation") are responded to with All-the-Way Opposite Action to reduce the emotion as quickly as possible. This is important to block Emotion Mind behavior as well as reduce subjective distress. The challenge in DBT Next Steps (vs. when they learned it in SDBT) is to really do All-the-Way Opposite Action. How to go above and beyond in Opposite Action should be explained and strongly encouraged. Emotions that are not effective often change to effective emotions once they are smaller, so it is frequently the case that both sets of skills will be required.

8. The flowchart (p. 120) illustrates how clients may need to move from Opposite Action around to Problem Solving or Mindfulness of Current Emotion. It is then reframed as a series of steps to work through as an example. Help the clients follow through the flowchart

in general and with a couple of examples of effective and ineffective emotions. For instance, to continue the example of the boss's criticism in a staff meeting, the client should first Check the Facts and decide if that is really the problem and what the primary emotion is—let's say, humiliation, with a SUDS of 85. Once facts are clear, determine if the humiliation is effective at that level and intensity. Let's say facts don't support that as it was a side comment and typical of bosses at staff meetings. So, the client practices Opposite Action and gets down the humiliation to embarrassment, at a SUDS of 45. The group leader might ask the client, "Is this emotion effective at the SUDS of 45 and its duration?" and decide it is. If they want to be more regulated, then the client might want to do Problem Solving or Mindfulness of Current Emotion (as noted in item 7a above) to work on how to respond to future critical comments.

9. Another example in a self-management context is being asked to go out with friends to dinner and a movie at the end of the month when money is tight. This might trigger an emotion of shame at 75. Check the Facts indicates that friends asked them to go out, but the dinner plus the movie was only a general idea and not a committed plan. So, the problem was restated as being asked to go out with friends, which could potentially cost more money than they had right now. Restating the facts brought the shame SUDS to 60. Mindful assessment tells the client that this is still higher than is effective in the situation. So, the client could practice Opposite Action by texting right back with humor that money is tight and they'd love it if something less inexpensive could be planned; otherwise, they'd catch them next time. This could bring SUDS down to 40, which would be evaluated as an effective emotion. If useful, Problem Solving could be applied to change the situation (find friends who are also broke to hang out with that night or plan to save money in a cookie jar for future end-of-the-month social activities) or their emotions about it (focus on how much debt they've paid off). Alternatively, the client could plan a Mindfulness of Current Emotion exercise for the next time such a text arrives.

Presenting the Week 2 Assignment

1. In the Week 2 Assignment: Regulating Yourself When You Need It, clients are asked to identify the top five problems/cues in work/school, social, and self-management contexts that dysregulate them (pp. 122–123).
2. Once this is completed (some people have to do this right away as their therapy session is the day after group), they show their list to their therapist who identifies their top five. These may be the same or different issues.
3. Remind clients that assessment tasks require Mindfulness skills. The clients should practice Mindfulness by activating curiosity, practicing describing rather than assuming or interpreting situations, and being nonjudgmental and effective in the process.
4. The next step of the Week 2 Assignment is to practice the in-class exercise three times this week on their own problems, selecting one from each key Recovery Goal context: work/school, social, and self-management (pp. 124–126).

5. The assignment cues the client to start early and give time for each task, as this is a difficult assignment for most clients to do well at the last minute.
6. Steps 1–4 are just like the example explored in group. Step 5 asks them to try acting on their plan. As noted, encourage clients to try and have the problem come up this week so they can test their plan while it is ready to go.
7. If clients express doubts about their ability to use the skills for that problem, remind them that they can do Cope Ahead imaginal rehearsal of their plan prior to a real situation arising.

Reviewing the Week 2 Assignment

1. The best way to efficiently review this assignment is to divide the whiteboard (or a shared document in telehealth) into three sections—work/school, social, and self-management—and have the clients list the problems they or their therapist came up with (that they are willing to share, as there may be some issues not appropriate to discuss a group context).
2. It is helpful to have the full list on the wall as it gives other clients the opportunity to add items to their own list they didn't think of. This should be encouraged if these issues are really top five issues (i.e., don't just create a long to-do list that includes nonimportant issues or reflects Emotion Mind perfectionism, rather than effectiveness and Wise Mind).
3. Ask clients if they observed interesting differences in what they identified and what their therapist identified. Have a discussion of perspective and the greater and lesser value of a second opinion of what is essentially a private experience.
4. For the second part of the assignment, it is unlikely that there will be time for all clients to review all three assignments. If there is, that is useful; however, it is also the case that after reviewing four to five examples, the relevant points have been highlighted and it becomes repetitious. Ask others to review their assignment for anything new or confusing and, if nothing comes up, move on.
5. Be sure to have at least one example from each context reviewed in class, as the issues involved in them can differ a lot.
6. Encourage additional examples that differ from those reviewed (e.g., effective vs. ineffective emotions, "changing the situation" solutions vs. "changing response to situations" solutions).
7. Be sure that the assignment is done correctly and that the Check the Facts part comes up with a problem that is described nonjudgmentally.
8. Be sure the solutions generated are fairly effective. Avoid accepting Problem-Solving solutions that seem ineffective or likely to cause new problems because group leaders accepting ineffective solutions can become quite confusing to other clients and suggests that the skills taught in this lesson are ineffective. If that was the only solution the client could generate, use the group to generate alternatives that would be more effective.
9. Reinforce determination, creativity, flexibility, and perseverance.

Week 3: Identifying and Managing Irritability

Key Points for Teaching

1. This lesson follows the sequence of first identifying the experience of irritability and assessing the contexts in which it arises, then problem solving (pp. 127–130).
2. Engage the group in describing their experience of irritability and getting specific with one example. Note the range of words in the handout for irritability (or its relations of "aggravation," "frustration," or "exasperation").
3. While defining irritability, stress the understanding in DBT Next Steps that Irritability = Irritants/Aversive sensations + Thoughts that it shouldn't be like this. Provide your own examples of this; describing them nonjudgmentally is key.
4. The "Only five possible responses to irritability" section (p. 130) draws from the "Options for Solving Any Problem" (General Handout 1A from SDBT; Linehan, 2025a, 2025b). It can prove useful to reference this handout to discuss how irritability might be solved in a similar way to other problems.

Presenting the Week 3 Assignment

1. As in previous weeks, the Week 3 Assignment starts with asking clients to track their experience of anger and irritability every day (p. 131). This is done from the perspective of their private experience and the reactions of others to their public behaviors. This is helpful for clients who do not have insight into how their anger and irritability affect those around them, and thus may not realize how irritable they are. The table offers a range of reactions that are cues they are being irritable even when others don't tell them outright.
2. Clients will then note their top 10 irritants (p. 132) as well as how they've stayed miserable or made it worse in the face of the irritants. It can be useful to clarify that staying miserable or making it worse generally happens outside of one's awareness, and that this exercise is about increasing awareness and insight.
3. To prepare clients to list examples for removing the irritant (p. 132), changing how you feel, and accepting/tolerating the irritant, encourage them to reference the examples listed in the handout under "Only five possible responses to irritability" (p. 130). The more concrete examples are, the better to provide group members with an understanding of how these methods are different.

Reviewing the Week 3 Assignment

1. Review the self-monitoring of anger and irritation (p. 131) as a group, asking everyone what their range of anger and irritation ratings were, what private experiences came up most, what public behaviors occurred, and what reactions from others resulted.
2. Have the clients take turns sharing their top 10 irritants. If anyone can't come up with 10, they may want to add irritants that other clients mention to their own list.
3. Review at least one irritant for each client. Focus on being precise and clear with the

categories of changing the situation, altering the way you feel, and accepting, so you don't confuse clients by accepting incorrect answers.

4. Reinforce participation, insight, willingness, and hope.

Week 4: Managing Anxiety with the Body and the Mind

Key Points for Teaching

1. This lesson starts with Progressive Muscle Relaxation (PMR) and then adds a cognitive strategy, the Four Questions to Manage Anxiety.
2. PMR is explained by David Barlow and Michelle Craske (2007). If group leaders are not familiar with PMR as a core element of anxiety treatments, they should review the panic control treatment workbook (Barlow & Craske, 2022) to understand exactly how body tension triggers anxiety and how PMR is critical to reducing this cue.
3. While PMR is part of SDBT TIPP skills, it is rarely practiced in SDBT in favor of the dive into ice water, intense exercise, or paced breathing, which are all easier to do when very dysregulated. PMR is often skipped over, but as it is critical to resolving anxiety, it is re-introduced here.
4. The scripts for PMR are provided along with some helpful tips (pp. 134–137). It is not expected that the scripts will be reviewed line for line, but the idea of moving from a 16-muscle group to cue PMR should be clarified. This is the gold-standard PMR process.
5. Group leaders should lead a 16-muscle-group PMR during group to provide an illustration and then hold a discussion afterward to address issues and concerns. Clients may want to audio-record this exercise so they have it to practice with during the week.
6. Next, introduce the Four Questions to Manage Anxiety with Your Mind handout (p. 138). This handout addresses interpretations by giving specific areas in which to "check the facts" and to be sure you are being anxious "correctly."
7. Note that the skills leader needs to stay accurate here and not minimize the client's anxiety or you will undercut your credibility on this skill. If things are really dangerous or terrible, you'll need to go to Question 4 to cope, rather than minimize Questions 1–3.
8. Highlight that the four questions have to be asked of Wise Mind, or at least Reasonable Mind (not Emotion Mind). If anxiety is too high, it might be necessary to do PMR, TIPP, or use some other strategy to clear the mind enough to find Wise Mind.
9. The questions are as follows:
   a. *"What is the worst thing that can happen?"* It is important not to minimize the real threat but to challenge worst-case scenarios that are, in fact, unrealistic catastrophes (i.e., so unrealistic the group will agree that it is) or tangential problems that aren't really related to the threat at hand (if the tangential issue turns out to be the key issue, then you may need to start over addressing that problem).
   b. *"How likely is it that the worst thing will actually occur?"* If the situation is actually very unlikely to occur and the individual can accept this, anxiety will naturally decline.

Again, stay accurate here; if it is likely, don't minimize that, as Questions c or d below are useful for likely events.

c. *"How bad would the worst thing actually be?"* The key here is to make the endpoints of the scale REALLY extreme—life-destroying, family-destroying events. This is central to putting events in perspective so that everything is not a disaster, only real disasters are. Examples include being raped and murdered, being imprisoned for the rest of your life, your child being killed, and so forth. We are trying to identify the extreme end of a continuum to force the specific situations the clients are likely to find themselves in and to fit those situations along the 1–10 continuum. Without explicit prompting for an extreme endpoint, most anxious clients will rate almost anything over 5 and rate a great many things as 10.

   i. Ask clients to give examples and challenge the worst things that aren't really the worst things that could happen to them.

   ii. Sometimes it can help to put other not-so-bad and really bad events from the individual's life on this scale so they can relate the anchors (1, 5, 10) to benchmarks from their own life. When the current worst-case scenario is rated lower than other bad things the client has survived or coped with (and certainly less than the extreme rating), their anxiety will decline.

d. *"What skills would you use or how would you cope if the worst thing did occur?"* The key here is to have details of skills, including an exit strategy or Plan B, C, or D. Be sure the plan is realistic—something the individual could pull off. Act as if this is a real worst-case scenario (not just anxiety) when planning what to do. With a strong coping plan, anxiety will decline.

   i. For example, a client was afraid someone would start shooting on her bus as many people on her route carried guns and would argue and fight. She came up with a plan for how she would get under the seat and how to exit the bus when she could.

   ii. If you come up with a minimal plan, you are unlikely to have real faith that the worst case can be survived and coped with so your anxiety will not go down.

   iii. The act of coping with the worst-case scenario as a valid thing to problem-solve and cope ahead for often validates the client's valid fears.

   iv. Invalid fears tend to fall apart when planning a coping plan. Sometimes it's pretty funny and everyone gets a good laugh.

Presenting the Week 4 Assignment

1. The first part of the Week 4 Assignment is to practice PMR twice a day (p. 139). Recommend maintaining the 16-muscle-group full practice until they rate over 70 on the scale of relaxation and concentration more than once. Then move to the 8-muscle-group practice, and so on.
2. Clients may prefer to use an existing PMR tape or app. This is often easier for them and will generalize well to their life after DBT Next Steps graduation, so it can be encouraged. However, if the client has great difficulty relaxing, they should pick a longer option (20–30

minutes) rather than a 5- or 9-minute option available in many apps. Also, clarify that you want them to do PMR specifically and not replace it with guided imagery or another relaxation induction. Note that some PMRs come with music that clients may find irritating, so they may want to look for an option without music or use their recording of the in-class practice.

3. Troubleshoot with the clients what could go wrong with doing PMR, as this homework is often avoided by DBT Next Steps clients. Who might avoid doing it and why? Try and problem-solve solutions and practice commitment strategies together before group is over.
4. Clients are asked to twice complete the Four Questions to Manage Anxiety with Your Thoughts for two scenarios (pp. 140–141):
   a. Current anxiety (either mild or serious, but something that is a current fear for them)
   b. Serious anxiety (either currently or one that has been serious in the past or will likely come up in the future)
5. Highlight for clients that it is time to complete a Self-Assessment of Recovery Goals (pp. 142–145). They should complete it and give it to their therapist, or bring it to group next week and the group leaders will pass it along to the individual therapist. Remind clients that the goal is to take stock of progress in DBT Next Steps and be sure that their individual therapy is on track.

Reviewing the Week 4 Assignment

1. Conduct a missing-links analysis if clients did not practice PMR twice a day. This is very important because the reasons they don't do it here will likely reflect why they haven't done it before and whether they do it in the future.
2. Discuss the experience of PMR. Who actually felt relaxed—ever, frequently? For those who did not observe relaxation, what did they observe? Provide feedback to address any concerns. If the client has anxiety and does not seem to have taken to this task, encourage them to do further problem solving in individual therapy because it can make or break whether they will be able to reduce their anxiety in the long run.
3. Review the Four Questions to Manage Anxiety with Your Thoughts and discuss which question led to anxiety reduction.
4. Discuss how they can use the Four Questions going forward.
5. If the clients brought their Self-Assessment of Recovery Goals to session (instead of giving it to their individual therapist), collect it and give to their individual therapist.

CHAPTER 19

Module: Succeeding after DBT

General Notes

1. This module is designed to help clients with the transition out of the DBT approach after they leave DBT Next Steps and to improve their success in whichever medical or behavioral health care they choose. The general structure of the module is to strengthen and generalize skills practice; to highlight therapy-interfering behaviors (TIBs) of clients and therapists that may have led to therapy failures or problems; and to teach clients about how to consider their treatment options after DBT Next Steps and the practice in how to be effective with usual-care psychotherapy and usual-care medical providers post DBT Next Steps, in case these services are used.
2. The key first point is that, consistent with the DBT Next Steps goal of self-sufficiency, we do *not* expect or particularly encourage clients to continue in psychosocial treatment after completing DBT Next Steps (or pharmacotherapy, unless they have found a psychotropic regimen that is effective for them with side effects that do not inhibit the learning capacity and energy they need to sustain a nondisabled life). The principle, which is articulated in the week 3 materials in this module, is that the combination of DBT and DBT Next Steps should provide the treatment and learning needed to manage their own emotions and behavior to keep themselves stable, employed, and involved in normative communities they like. Especially in DBT Next Steps with the Recovery Goals, Check-In, and contingencies, the treatment is designed to teach clients to be their own therapist and case manager.
3. That being said, many clients have issues beyond basic management of their life for which they could use psychotherapeutic assistance. For instance, many clients have comorbid anxiety disorders (e.g., PTSD, generalized anxiety disorder [GAD], obsessive–compulsive disorder [OCD]) that are not entirely resolved by DBT or DBT Next Steps and for which they might want specialized care. Life events and transitions occur, and in response, the client might benefit from psychotherapy (e.g., divorce, loss, moving to a new state, having children, empty nest). Other clients might have DBT "Stage 4" questions about how they

came to have the problems they did and want to pursue some insight-oriented treatment, or perhaps they could use some assistance in managing the grief they experience in the tragedies of their life that they haven't resolved. Thus, future treatment should be articulated throughout this module (and DBT Next Steps) as a dialectical tension between recognition and adapting to their own capacity to care for themselves, and recognition and acceptance of specific areas where therapeutic care would be effective. However, it should *not* be conveyed to DBT Next Steps clients in general (such as in group) that they are expected to need treatment after DBT Next Steps.

4. Whether or not clients want or need behavioral health care following DBT Next Steps, they are likely to be involved in other health care such as primary care, gynecology, obstetrics, physical therapy, and so forth. Many of the principles in this module have applications to medical and other health care, and this should also be highlighted.
5. Building on the prior points, it is critical that the DBT Next Steps individual therapists and group leaders have exiting long-term mental health programs clearly in mind as these clients' goal (which in the United States implies not receiving treatment in the public mental health system, which includes disability as an eligibility criterion). Doubt in the mind of the therapists will escalate clients' fears of leaving long-term programs and is not helpful.
6. On the other hand, this module is designed to highlight specific skills the clients will need to master before the end of DBT Next Steps if they are to succeed outside of long-term programs. Examples have included hopeless thinking, passivity, in-session TIBs, lack of insurance, lack of funds for outside therapy or medications if they need them, and the like. Group leaders should emphasize not that these aren't reasons to remain in long-term mental health programs, but rather they are the key issues that the DBT Next Steps group and the client and their individual therapist will need to focus on for the remainder of DBT Next Steps. Much of this focus is carried by the individual therapist, as it is only addressed in group as part of this module and sometimes as it relates to Check-In.
7. While this module is critical of standard public mental health services as a long-term plan for clients with BPD graduating from DBT, that is not to say these services aren't quite valuable to many other clients. It is generally helpful to have the DBT consultation team discuss these handouts and the implications prior to starting this module to be sure that everyone understands and agrees with the DBT Next Steps philosophy therein.
8. Note also, this is an area in which time in DBT Next Steps plays an obvious role. Clients who are early in DBT Next Steps tend to panic at the idea of graduating from DBT Next Steps and not going on to another psychotherapist or case manager. They will say clearly that they will not be able to do this. By contrast, many of those completing a second 6 months of DBT Next Steps in a 1-year program are often relieved to talk about the end of DBT. Much like an adolescent being ready to fly out of the nest, many clients approaching a year in DBT Next Steps will be more in the "I'm ready to get out of here" phase (even if they like the treatment). It can be helpful to highlight this difference and the natural development that occurs over two 6-month rounds of DBT Next Steps.
9. Some DBT Next Steps clients and programs will only last 6 months and travel through these handouts only once. It is likely that the types of clients who are only doing DBT Next Steps for 6 months will be more ready to complete treatment and move onto the next stage of their

life. If someone is having a major anxiety response, this should be addressed in individual therapy and, if justified anxiety, a second round of DBT Next Steps should be considered.

10. It is important to note that this module involves the individual therapist and potentially the pharmacotherapist.
    a. The clients should be alerted to this so they can discuss assignments with their individual therapists ahead of weeks 2, 3, and 4.
    b. If they want to plan for their medications with their pharmacotherapist in week 3 (part of the assignment on p. 159), then they may want to call and schedule an appointment for that week ahead of this module.
    c. Group leaders may also want to alert individual therapists in a DBT consult meeting, so therapists who may be focused on other issues have time to fit this content into this month's sessions.
    d. In the 1-year version of DBT Next Steps when the clients will experience this module twice, it can be helpful to do the role-plays in week 4 with the pharmacotherapist on the second time through, rather than repeating with the individual therapist, or do both. This is probably too much for clients in the first of two rounds of DBT Next Steps skills, but the individual therapist might decide to include the pharmacotherapist as well on a case-by-case basis.
    e. If someone will need to change pharmacotherapists at the end of the DBT Next Steps program, it can be helpful to arrange this change during DBT Next Steps, rather than at the end—another reason for engaging the current or a new prescriber on the first of two rounds of DBT Next Steps skills. Psychiatric clinicians are often more comfortable taking on a client while they are in therapy and deciding with the client whether they will be ready to become the sole person managing the case after DBT Next Steps or if they need the client to have a psychosocial provider as well. In the latter situations, it is ideal if a client can meet with an individual therapist for a brief period after DBT Next Steps to forge a relationship and future plan. Then the client would not attend that therapy regularly, but has the therapist in the background if an issue comes up. We have found this a good synthesis of the needs of a psychiatrist with a very large panel of patients who is unwilling to take sole clinical responsibility and our DBT Next Steps goal that we don't fragilize clients who can function without ongoing therapy.

Week 1: Practice DBT 24/7

Key Points for Teaching

1. The primary idea here is that clients vary tremendously in the amount of DBT focus they bring to their life. Some bring a focus on DBT and skills only in the difficult moments. Others focus most of the time but give up when the going gets really rough. Others have gotten so good at their DBT skills, they stop using them mindfully and just count on the ones they've overlearned to do the job. These strategies may be fine in many instances, but they are probably not going to work during the difficult moments when the clients are on their own after graduating from DBT Next Steps. The idea is to teach them how to bring that focus all the time, if and when needed.

2. Note that we are not saying, "From this day forward you will do DBT 24/7 for the rest of your life." We are saying that it is an experience to practice DBT so fully, and we want them to have that experience. At many times in their life, it will not be necessary to do DBT 24/7, but everyone has a time when their back is to the wall and they need to be able to do every skill in every way for a good long time. This practice is to teach them what it is like and what DBT 24/7 can offer to them. Encourage the clients to throw themselves into the practice for this 1 week and not get too attached to whether they will ever do it again.
3. Complete the Practice DBT 24/7 handout with the clients in class (p. 149). Walk them through answering Questions 1–6, stopping to discuss any points as needed. The assignment this week presumes this has already been done.
4. This is primarily a commitment strategy handout designed to set the stage for clients to do DBT 24/7 for a full week. It can be very helpful to have each client pick a strategy in Question 6 and then have the group leaders talk about how they would use it to increase their number in Question 5. This is what they will have to do as part of their assignment this week, and sometimes they don't really understand how to use the strategies. Having each one illustrated with a different client helps make the strategies clearer.
5. Group leaders should frame the nature of commitment to practicing skills (and any other behavior change) as fluid rather than fixed. That is, consider how level of commitment might change moment to moment, responding to the context that a client is in. For example, commitment to practicing PLEASE might be easier while spending the day with a friend who values "taking care of the body to take care of the mind," compared to spending the day with a friend who doesn't exercise or eat healthily and is defensive about it. Commitment can be similar to turning-the-mind, in that we are planning for times when we might fight with reality and are making an inner commitment to turning our mind toward acceptance.
6. Emphasize that to achieve DBT 24/7, it is important to actively plan for the factors that will get in the way of our commitment and problem-solve to enhance our commitment. Group leaders can draw from Self-Management Recovery Goals for examples (see Chapter 4 for a detailed discussion of these Recovery Goals).

Presenting the Week 1 Assignment

1. Orient the clients that the in-class discussion will now continue as the at-home Week 1 Assignment: Practice DBT 24/7 (p. 150). If you have time, you can do Questions 1 and 2 during class.
2. Use extending strategies, irreverence, or whatever you need to get the clients to really buy into the idea that they will use DBT skills every minute for 1 week.
3. Remind clients (especially the perfectionists in the room) that this is NOT your expectation of what they will do forever from this day forward. It is instead designed as an experience for them to try and expose themselves to the idea of doing skills all the time.
4. The key is for them to see what is the same or different between DBT 24/7 and their typical way of doing DBT skills, and how differently they might have experienced the two approaches. They should write down these observations in Question 4.
5. Right before group, they should complete Question 5.

Reviewing the Week 1 Assignment

1. First, ask each client to trace their commitment to DBT 24/7 from Question 5 on the in-class handout to Question 2 on the weekly assignment, and then to Question 5 on the assignment. Practice curiosity. Did it increase, decrease, stay the same? What, if anything, was a surprise to them?
2. Review which strategies they picked in response to Question 1 on the assignment, how they planned to use them, and how they actually used them. Reinforce effort, persistence, flexibility, and creativity. If they didn't use the strategies, conduct a missing-links analysis, as this is an important part of the exercise.
3. Review their observations from Question 4. Validate difficulty and reinforce effort, persistence, flexibility, and creativity.

Week 2: Therapy-Interfering Behavior

Key Points for Teaching

1. The goal of this week's lesson is to bring to clients' awareness the idea of therapy-interfering behavior (TIB) and allow them to consider where it has been a problem for them in their treatment history. It addresses both their TIB and the TIB of previous therapists (including in SDBT and DBT Next Steps).
2. Because not all participants in DBT Next Steps have borderline personality disorder (BPD), the module refers throughout to "problems of emotion regulation, interpersonal sensitivity, or distress tolerance."
3. This is a time to remember the DBT case management guidelines in terms of not defending other providers (even if they are on your DBT team), while at the same time keeping everyone in Describe language (no judgments, assumptions, and interpretations). It can be helpful to highlight when Describe skills are needed.
4. Note, you can teach and use the phrase "What makes you say that?" as a way to cue others to use Describe skills (i.e., behaviorally specific language), utilizing language that's normative for conversation. This is a nice option for clients to use with friends and family who continue to be judgmental without directly asking them to be nonjudgmental, which is often not a welcome request.
5. This is also a time for radical genuineness about the clients' TIBs and to highlight for them the TIBs that could in any way jeopardize their ability to succeed with a typical therapist or other health care provider. Better for them to hear this now—from the group leaders and individual therapist—rather than pay a price for it later from clinicians who may not be genuine about why the client is being fired.
6. On the other hand, this does not mean we should go around the room calling out clients' failings. Instead, the DBT Next Steps materials will encourage them to recognize TIBs, and the group leaders and therapists can endorse what they see as valid. If there are other TIBs the client does not see, the materials provide an opportunity for the individual therapist to raise them with the client privately, and the group leaders can use their clinical judgment about what to bring up in group.

7. Review the Therapy-Interfering Behaviors handout (pp. 151–154) during group. Go through the lists of problems in previous treatment in a nonjudgmental fashion and encourage clients to add additional problems.
8. The goal here is to help clients understand that the problems they have are (a) typical of therapy with clients who struggle with emotion regulation, interpersonal sensitivity, and distress tolerance in general, not themselves personally; (b) as much a limitation of the therapists and treatments available for problems of emotion regulation, interpersonal sensitivity, and distress tolerance as of clients themselves; and (c) likely to re-occur.
9. It should be highlighted that DBT is a unique treatment in that it has many skills and strategies built in to manage TIBs of emotionally dysregulated clients, which most therapists don't have or don't use.
10. This is the beginning of teaching the notion that therapy after DBT should only be for a specific area for which the new therapist is an expert. As an expert in another area, the new therapist cannot be expected to also be an expert in DBT, BPD, or problems of emotion regulation, interpersonal sensitivity, and distress tolerance as well.
11. Pages 151–154 of this handout are taken primarily from material on TIBs in Marsha Linehan's DBT treatment manual (Linehan, 1993, pp. 131–137), with some additions from DBT Next Steps clients who completed this module. For these handouts, group leaders can read the items aloud or go around the room, with each person naming one TIB and everyone checking off those that apply to them or their treatment experience. Clients should be encouraged to add additional behaviors.

Presenting the Week 2 Assignment

1. The Week 2 Assignment is based on further consideration of the prior handout—first by the client on their own, then by interviewing their individual therapist (and others as makes sense). The goal is to generate their "top 10" list of remaining TIBs for themselves that the individual therapist and client will commit to changing during the course of DBT Next Steps (p. 155).
2. The tone of this discussion with the individual therapist and in group must differ for clients depending on where they are in the DBT Next Steps process. Since this module can come up for clients at any time during DBT Next Steps, graduation might seem far away and not that relevant if they are on an urgent job search at the beginning, and it can feel as if there is not nearly enough time left to deal with this when they are at the end. Individual therapists and group leaders should use their clinical judgment and dialectical strategies to manage this tension.
3. Clients (and therapists) can draw from the assessments done as part of the comprehensive DBT ACES program application to get a reminder of previous TIBs. Revisiting the client's DBT-ACES application is one option to consider when completing this assignment.

Reviewing the Week 2 Assignment

1. The review of this assignment is straightforward—have clients report on a few examples of their TIBs that they are willing to share.

2. Sometimes the "team" of group leaders and other DBT Next Steps clients agree to work together to help the client overcome that problem (e.g., by highlighting the problem when it arises or blocking it), but group leaders should use clinical judgment based on their group's makeup and the issue as to when to encourage this. In some cases, this has been extremely effective. For instance, reassurance seeking is a common TIB for our clients, particularly those with GAD for whom getting reassurance neutralizes (temporarily) their worry thoughts and anxiety. This can ultimately be unhelpful to them. DBT Next Steps groups have been helpful in joining together in a good-humored plan to block reassurance seeking. Other clients may be better at noticing the behaviors that function as reassurance seeking than the group leaders, making it easier for them to block it with a kind or humorous cue, allowing the DBT Next Steps group to be nonreinforced exposure for the client. Judgments and self-invalidation are other TIBs the "team" of DBT Next Steps clients and group leaders can work together to highlight and block. That being said, groups differ and clinical judgment is needed to determine when this will be helpful.
3. Note, if clients do not complete the interview with their individual therapist due to timing or other key therapy issues that the individual therapist prioritized instead, the client should be clearly directed to get it done as soon as possible and report back to the co-leader when it is completed. This is a critical lesson in DBT Next Steps and should not be allowed to slip by.

Week 3: Your Future and Therapy

Key Points for Teaching

1. The goal of this lesson is to think through options for care following DBT Next Steps. The handouts reflect a combination of the DBT Next Steps philosophy, health services research, and clinical observations of previous DBT Next Steps clients. The goal is to educate clients about the less obvious implications of their treatment choices so they can make more effective decisions.
2. A core DBT Next Steps perspective is that the Check-In, Recovery Goal, Work as Therapy, Diary Card, and self-assessments, as well as the DBT Next Steps Skills Curriculum and individual therapy, are all focused on the client becoming able to manage their own behavior without the need for a psychotherapist, case manager, family, and the like. This is discussed by the individual therapist as treatment goes along and is part of the interview in the DBT-ACES pretreatment process for those using the comprehensive program. And, it is important to call it out here. As noted above, being without a therapist or other support provider is often quite alarming for new DBT Next Steps clients, but much more reasonable to DBT Next Steps clients nearing graduation. It is important that group leaders convey confidence in such a plan as they teach this material.
3. If leaders have concerns about this plan for DBT Next Steps clients after graduation, in general or as it applies to a given client, it is important to address this in the consultation team before teaching this module.
4. For some clients with the financial means or insurance to pay for it, having a psychotherapist for the long run (DBT or otherwise) can be helpful. However, it is not recommended

they remain in therapy. An alternative is to see a new therapist for a short period (maybe 2–4 months) to get to know the therapist and obtain some assistance in beginning their post-DBT Next Steps life. After this transition, they can taper or stop regular therapy sessions and set up a long-term plan to return if and when needed for booster sessions or help if they hit a snag (e.g., lose a job or have another kind of life transition). Thus, they are using the therapist as they would a primary care provider: someone who is around and available, seen for check-ups, but otherwise fades into the background.

5. Review the options for treatment after DBT Next Steps (pp. 156–157) as a group. Encourage client examples and coach for nonjudgmental descriptions of their hopes and concerns. Correct any inaccurate understandings that clients might have about any treatment option.
6. At the end of the handout (p. 157), clients are told to "Consider the websites and resources provided by your therapists for finding and evaluating treatment options." Given that behavioral health services differ around the world and change over time, specific handouts are not provided for this. The DBT Next Steps team should put together their best materials on where to find clinicians, online/smartphone or other treatment options, and the "how-to's" of evaluating treatment quality (e.g., How to interview a therapist? How to evaluate their credentials? How to know if an app has been tested?).
7. Review the next handout, Being the Best Client You Can Be to Get the Best Care (p. 158), by asking everyone to read an option, or having clients read it to themselves and highlight any items they question or disagree with for discussion. Some of these standards are quite high, but since most DBT Next Steps clients can meet them, they may as well have such standards as a goal. The mission here is to help clients understand and practice radical acceptance for the limits of psychotherapy. They can't just attend psychotherapy and expect that to be enough to get what they need.
8. It should be noted that the same can be said for health care generally, and this should be highlighted for clients who do not plan to continue in behavioral health care after DBT Next Steps.
9. Group leaders may want to give clients useful questions to ask when picking a DBT therapist or program (adapted from Linda Dimeff and Portland DBT Institute, 2014):
   a. Are you on a DBT consultation team? If yes, what percentage of your DBT team has been intensively/comprehensively trained by a recognized DBT expert?
   b. Do clients in the program do Diary Cards?
   c. Do you routinely audio-/video-record your DBT individual therapy sessions, and does your DBT team listen to and critique each other's sessions to make sure you are engaged in adherent therapy?
   d. Do you offer all of the following elements of comprehensive DBT?
      i. DBT individual therapy (1 hour weekly)
      ii. DBT skills-training class (typically, 2 hours weekly)
      iii. DBT consultation team (1 hour per week for clinicians)
      iv. Out-of-session coaching (as needed, provided by the individual therapist)
   e. Available during or outside of standard work hours?

Presenting the Week 3 Assignment

1. The Week 3 Assignment: Your Future and Therapy (p. 159) requires discussion with the individual therapist as well as any pharmacotherapist. The assignment is to think through plans for treatment following DBT Next Steps (if any) and to talk this through with the DBT therapist and pharmacotherapist.
2. The goal here is to maximize client gains and minimize the risk of a treatment program that reinforces maladaptive behavior or otherwise triggers a relapse to "dependency behavior."
3. This assignment has different meaning for clients who are early versus late in DBT Next Steps, so clients should be reminded to be effective in terms of this assignment and their time in DBT Next Steps.
4. Note that many patients have simplified and stabilized their medications since joining DBT and are no longer in need of a psychiatrist, so their care could be transferred to a primary care provider. This will be something that varies by health system, so the only DBT Next Steps recommendation is to focus on what works for the client. That being said, we have found that making a transfer of pharmacotherapy while the client is in DBT Next Steps and having access to weekly psychotherapy are more reassuring to a pharmacotherapist new to the client or the primary care provider taking over their psychotropic medications. To that end, if DBT Next Steps clients expect to experience a change in pharmacotherapy after DBT (e.g., from a psychiatrist to primary care provider or from a prescriber who is part of the DBT clinic to someone independent), we encourage them to make this transfer fairly early in DBT Next Steps so the prescriber has support while they get to know the client. This often leads to them being happy to continue with the client without psychotherapy after DBT Next Steps is concluded. Alternatively, after working together, the prescriber may be clear that they will require the client to attend some form of behavioral health treatment so the prescriber remains willing to continue prescribing after DBT Next Steps graduation. In the case of the latter, the DBT Next Steps client and therapist have time to work on such a plan prior to the termination of treatment.

Reviewing the Week 3 Assignment

1. Much of the decision making here is deferred to the individual therapist and pharmacotherapist, so the group leaders are generally fairly neutral and reflective in review of this homework so as not to complicate matters.
2. Conduct missing-links analysis if the client avoids completing this assignment.
3. Reinforce ambition, hope, interpersonal effectiveness, and finding Wise Mind.

Week 4: Practice Making Non-DBT Treatment Work

Key Points for Teaching

1. This week is focused on how to communicate with providers about information in the client's medical record (or other clinical information) that could cause concern for non-DBT providers (pp. 160–161). When teaching this skill, consider determining a script of what

to say in the first part, and then role-playing in class as the second part, leading into the homework assignment, which is to generalize by role-playing with the individual therapist (and/or pharmacotherapist).

2. Group leaders will want to set the stage by highlighting scenarios that involve a new provider's concern and a client's skillful attempts at alleviating the concerns:
   a. A common scenario has been that the client says they are having suicidal thoughts, and the therapist reacts by saying they have to go to the emergency room (ER) instead of working on the problem that led to the suicidal ideation. For the role play, the group leader or another client should be the therapist with this concern and the client should practice strategies to effectively assure the therapist that the risk of suicide is not imminent. The person playing the therapist might persist in wanting the client to go to the ER, so the client can persist in effectively reassuring the therapist until the group as a whole believes the client has been convincing.
   b. A TIB example (from week 2 of this module) would be the client grows quiet and the therapist becomes soothing and drops their demands. Thus, the client could role-play two things: being less quiet and showing more attentive nonverbals, and asking the therapist not to back off when they get quiet as that is not helpful, but rather to soothe when they are being successful.
3. It is often useful to role-play how not to say inflammatory things (like indirect suicide threats) or respond with defensiveness to doctors. Role plays provide an opportunity to increase exposure to these cues, which can sometimes be invalidating, prompt anger and ineffective urges, and create room for clients to proceed skillfully. Rather than just conveying their plan to remain stable on an outpatient plan, this skill is also an opportunity to attend to a new therapeutic relationship with GIVE skills (albeit one where several approaches in DBT might be missing, such as a nonjudgmental attitude and creating a balanced power equilibrium).
4. It is quite helpful to have a guest who is a prescriber or non-DBT therapist attend to play the clinician in these role plays. This adds to both the credibility and real-life feeling of the practice.
5. The leaders should consider ways to set up role plays of appointments going wrong and have the clients practice alternative strategies by linking the types of problems that each client has had with previous providers (Questions 1–3 from week 2) to their plan for their care after DBT Next Steps (from week 3).
6. With regard to suicide risk, clients will face barriers from their medical record or explaining their history while engaging a therapist with the expertise the client is looking for (in addition to a likely waitlist). Sometimes, it is strategic to choose a new therapist who doesn't share an electronic health record with clinicians who have seen and documented the client in crisis. This can be particularly important when the record has been unkind or otherwise unhelpfully describes the client and gives a negative impression. However, hiding history doesn't lead to a genuine and committed relationship.
7. We have found the most effective way to convince a clinician to take our clients on, or that they do not need to go to an ER or seek a higher level of care, is for the client to describe the skills that they will use to prevent or stop a dark moment so as not to harm or kill themself.

This involves showing the therapist a safety or crisis response plan, and clarifying what skills are Plan A and then what skills would be Plan B, Plan C, and so forth.

8. In the role plays regarding suicide or self-injury risk, the client practices describing a wide range of skills to cope and what skills they will use next. That is, providing reassurance to the therapist that the client is in the position to prevent and to get through a crisis. Essentially, the more skills, the more likely the therapist is reassured that there are ways by which the clients can independently work through it, and the therapist's anxiety about working with this client is likely to subside.
9. For suicidal behavior, it can also be helpful to describe reasons for living and why they outweigh reasons for dying. Clients can describe whom their suicide will harm and why they wouldn't risk that.
10. Consider the other side of appearing confident and in control of your life and the crisis: Therapists are often responsive to individuals who are open to their ideas/interpretations/suggestions. Many therapists are independent types and like having a lot of room to do things their way! Group leaders can engage the group in this dialectic—how to be independent in listing skills and being responsive to the strategies that the non-DBT therapist will suggest. Try engaging the group in identifying the skills that convey appearing confident (e.g., Appear Confident from DEAR MAN) as well as open and responsive to the therapist (e.g., Act Interested from GIVE)
11. DBT skills group has a guideline that suicidal behaviors are not explicitly discussed, and this is the one skills module where suicide and self-harm behaviors are talked about openly in group. It can be helpful for group leaders to acknowledge why this module is different; that is, to highlight the goal to increase interpersonal effectiveness around how to communicate with a non-DBT provider on issues relating to suicide risk. It requires clients to talk about the behaviors in clear and direct ways, and consider the perspective of their new treatment team.
12. Consider modeling before the client starts the role plays. Share the following script of DEAR MAN, or some variation, and include it if no other clients jump in with similar content during the discussion before the role plays:
    - D: "I want to discuss something that is in my chart, and that you might know about my history, and that is that I have a history of multiple suicide attempts and hospitalizations."
    - E: "I'd like to talk with you more about how I've learned to manage self-harm since learning skills in DBT."
    - A: "I have a range of DBT skills and strategies that have been useful for me when I start struggling, and I was hoping to go over some of them with you at some point to see what you think, and also get ideas about anything you might want to add to my ways of coping."
    - R: "I'm hoping that sharing this info will help us be on the same page about how to respond, since I really want this treatment to go well."

Presenting the Week 4 Assignment

1. The Week 4 Assignment: Practice Making Non-DBT Treatment Work (p. 162) involves clients choosing two situations that have been problematic for them historically (see the Week 2 Assignment) and role-playing how to handle them more effectively.

2. If the person has a history of suicide risk or self-harm, one of the role plays should be explicitly about that. If there is a history of violence, this should also be role-played, but it may be reviewed only with the individual therapist and not the group, depending on the context and the clinical judgment of the group leaders.
3. The second role play (or both role plays if there is no history of life-threatening behavior) should be from the list of top 10 TIBs from week 2 and not suicidal behavior. It is quite a different thing to role-play not doing a TIB and talking about not reinforcing TIB so that deserves its own practice.
4. Note, the client can do this role play with their therapist or others as long as the other person understands DBT Next Steps concepts sufficiently to provide a useful partner and give useful feedback afterward. For instance, some clients have explained the whole task to a previous provider and had them role-play or role-played with a friend who also is or was in DBT Next Steps.
5. As noted earlier, if this is the client's second time through the DBT Next Steps skills, it may be more valuable to have the client practice with their pharmacotherapist or primary care provider rather than their therapist again.
6. Highlight for clients that they need to make this work even if something goes wrong with Plan A for role playing. They should do some troubleshooting in group to assure their therapist saves enough time or schedule an extra session or whatever is needed to get this done this week. Of course, if they don't get the task done, this becomes a top priority to complete and the co-leader should be told when it has been completed.
7. Remind clients that they should provide their own observations as well as asking their role-play partner for their observations.

Reviewing the Week 4 Assignment

1. Use your clinical judgment and the considerations from teaching point 11 listed above about whether to review the suicidal behavior role plays in group. Generally, we have found that since DBT Next Steps clients haven't been suicidal for some time, this goes smoothly with a focus on how suicide is no longer an issue for them and their reasons for living, so there is a minimal risk of contagion. However, group leaders might choose to direct the clients to discuss that one with their individual therapist and avoid more explicit talk about suicidal behaviors in group.
2. Definitely review the TIB role plays in group and discuss both the clients' and their role-play partners' observations.
3. Depending on time and content, it can be useful to re-enact the TIB role plays in group if clients express an interest in how a client pulled something off, or if the role-play assignment didn't work out well.

CHAPTER 20

Module: Applications of Mindfulness

General Notes

1. There are two main foci of the DBT Next Steps application of Mindfulness skills: using mindfulness to manage problem thoughts and using mindfulness to increase acceptance.
2. The goal is for clients to incorporate mindfulness into their daily lives at a more profound and complete level than is often achieved after SDBT.
3. SDBT does not require the regular mindfulness practice of clients. However, in this module of DBT Next Steps, we have clients practice mindfulness each day for two reasons: (a) to provide them with an opportunity to try a daily practice, which has been extremely helpful for some clients, and (b) the mindfulness practice offers a chance to experience problematic thoughts and noticeable urges to change/avoid a situation and to practice accepting and experiencing it instead.
4. Note that daily mindfulness is a focus of this module. If the group leaders and individual therapists of the DBT Next Steps clients do not have a daily mindfulness practice (or haven't practiced daily for some time), they should practice at least a month of daily mindfulness prior to this module being taught in session so they can understand what that experience requires and is like, and be able to effectively assist clients to succeed.

Week 1: Daily Mindfulness Practice and Mindfulness to Control Attention

Key Points for Teaching

1. The first handout in the module (p. 165) orients clients to the plan of a daily mindfulness practice.
2. During the first 2 weeks of the module, clients can practice different mindfulness exercises

from any source. During the second 2 weeks of the module, clients will pick a mindfulness exercise and stay with it for the full 2 weeks.

3. Mindfulness exercises have the best effect if practiced regularly over time (daily practice over months or years). Duration of mindfulness exercises is less important than frequency—that is, doing them more often as opposed to longer.
   a. Emphasize the dialectic between a mindfulness practice that is too long (and that they avoid doing) versus one that is too short (and that they do not benefit from). Encourage clients to find a synthesis using shaping concepts to choose a duration where they have at least a 50% chance of achieving but it is not too easy for them.
   b. This could be 2 minutes, 5 minutes, 20 minutes, or an hour. They should commit to a time each day for the first 2 weeks, but if they need to reduce the time to get the exercise done, they should do so. For the second 2 weeks, however, they should commit to the specified duration and use their skills to pull it off.
   c. Clients often expect that mindfulness will (or "should" be) this peaceful moment and that a problem exists if mindfulness is distressing or difficult. Correct this misunderstanding and highlight that a major goal of this DBT Next Steps module is for them to learn how to use mindfulness to be mindful of distress (if it arises) and accept discomfort rather than avoid it.
   d. Remind them that they may have stopped using mindfulness practice in the past when it was not pleasant. We do not want them to stop as they practice at their daily scheduled time. It is through continuing to practice that the brain figures out how to stay with whatever comes (or doesn't).
4. Next, orient clients to the Mindfulness to Control Attention handout (pp. 166–167).
5. Clarify the meaning of "rumination" and "worry" and come up with examples.
6. Help clients understand why they ruminate and obsess even though it is often unpleasant and may even be ruining their lives (e.g., it feels as if they are working on a problem, avoidance of the moment or other difficult things, avoidance of something new).
7. Generate client examples of negative consequences of rumination, worry, and obsession (you can relate to the punishment strategy from the Perfectionism versus Reinforcement module, if they have completed it).
8. Help clients understand how mindfulness is incompatible with rumination or obsession (the equivalent of Training an Incompatible Behavior from the Perfectionism versus Reinforcement module).
9. Orient clients to the "Three Mindfulness Strategies," which are mindfulness alternatives to rumination and worry:
   a. *Mindfulness Exercise:* Doing a specific and different one-mindful action for an explicit period of time. Exercises might range from taking three deep, mindful breaths to a mindful walk, to a meditation. The idea is for the client to do something that brings mindfulness that is outside their current activities—a break from the rumination/obsession—to clear their mind and then return more effectively to the next moment.
   b. *One-Mindful Action:* Doing what is most effective in the moment, and doing it with all

of your attention. Instead of taking their mind to a mindfulness exercise outside the current moment, the client brings 100% one-mindful attention to the present moment and fully participates in what this moment calls for (do the thing that is scheduled at this time, finish the task they are doing, etc.)

c. *Mindful Assessment:* Considering a situation or what is best to do with Observe and Describe skills, one-mindfully and without judgment. The goal here is for the client to think about what they are ruminating on in a way that is actually useful and will get them to act effectively, as opposed to rumination or obsession, which goes in circles and leads to avoidance, poor decisions, and staying miserable. This is the right approach if there might actually be something to figure out, rather than their rehearsing what they already know. Often mindful assessment requires writing down something or discussing it with a friend or therapist—the line between mindful assessment and rumination/obsession can get blurry for people if done in their head. Clients who are big ruminators or obsessive can quickly move from mindful assessment to rumination/obsession, ending up back where they started. Having a partner or seeing it on paper can make a big difference in staying mindful.

d. *Example:* Sitting on the couch and ruminating about the breakup with your girlfriend. A mindfulness exercise might be counting your breath for 5 minutes. A mindful action might be to do what is most effective in that moment if you weren't ruminating (e.g., call a friend, watch TV, clean the house). Mindful assessment might involve nonjudgmentally writing out for yourself the situation with your girlfriend, what the likely future of the relationship is, and what your options are.

Presenting the Week 1 Assignment

1. The first task here will be the "Daily Mindfulness Practice" (p. 168).
2. Second, the Week 1 Assignment: Mindfulness to Control Attention handout requires careful orientation.
   a. First, you want clients to think about the roles rumination and obsession play in their life.
      i. Clients identify contexts in which they ruminate or obsess, such as locations (on the couch, in bed, on the bus, at my mother's house) or circumstances (when I'm alone, after being given negative feedback, near my birthday, when no one talks to me at social events, when I'm supposed to be working or trying to finish a paper for class).
      ii. Clients identify topics or subjects about which they tend to ruminate or obsess (my past, traumatic events, my future, my health, the quality of my work, whether people like me, whether I did things correctly, why I haven't gotten farther in my life by now, what is wrong with me).
   b. Next, they will practice responding with mindfulness instead of continuing to ruminate or obsess. Choosing one of the Three Mindfulness Strategies to respond means picking either (1) Mindfulness Exercise, (2) One-Mindful Action, or (3) Mindful Assessment. They should first pick one and then come up with a specific way they will do it.
   c. Remind clients that rumination, worry, and obsession are usually well under way before

they realize they are doing any of them. To block rumination and obsession, it is necessary to have a cue that reminds them to observe if they are ruminating or obsessing.

  i. The cue should occur *without* the client causing it in the moment because when they are ruminating or obsessing, they are unlikely to think to do anything. The cue is something that just happens naturally as they go through the day, which can serve as a periodic reminder to practice.
  ii. The idea is whenever the cue occurs (e.g., the client sees a string tied around their finger, hears a phone ring, hears their pet roaming around the house, or they come to a red stoplight while driving), the client observes whether they are ruminating or obsessing. If not, they can just go on with their day. If yes, then they should practice the Mindful Strategy they chose to replace the ruminating or obsessing.
  iii. Possible cues include tying a string on your finger (an oldie but goodie); wearing a different ring, watch, or bracelet that you will notice is different when it catches your eye; setting an alarm on your phone; buying a digital watch that gives reminders every hour; or using the ringing or a notification on your phone.
  iv. The cue should also be relevant to the contexts in which the client ruminates or worry, or it won't be effective. For example, if they don't ruminate or worry in the car, then using stoplights as a cue won't be very helpful.
  v. Have clients generate a range of viable cues during group, and they can decide on a cue at the end or after group.

d. Orient them to the plan to practice at least three times a day and note their observations about it. The key is that the cue has to occur at least three times per day, but shouldn't occur so often that it will overwhelm the client.

e. Use commitment and troubleshooting strategies as needed.

Reviewing the Week 1 Assignment

1. Be sure to review homework to practice daily mindfulness to (a) reinforce the notion that it must be done each day (do missing-links analysis and troubleshoot if this is not happening) and (b) troubleshoot any problems the clients are having with their practice.
2. Have clients describe one of their daily mindfulness practices.
3. Reinforce any positive experiences or insights as well as perseverance in doing the practice frequently. Reinforce effective and nonjudgmental problem solving.
4. Regarding the Three Mindfulness Strategies, have each client walk through what their specific mindful strategy was, what their cue was, and then find out how this worked. When/how was mindfulness able to successfully replace rumination and obsession? How long did it last? Did willfulness interfere? Did anxiety or shame interfere? What did the client like about it?
5. Highlight commonalities and differences between clients' experiences and troubleshoot problems.
6. Be alert that the mindfulness to control attention assignment is often done casually with no specific cue chosen or done on the fly, rather than with deliberation. If that is the case,

highlight that this is not an effective way to respond to assignments at work or school and the problems they may have with using these skills in a difficult moment if they have only practiced in a casual way.

Week 2: Opening and Refocusing the Mind

Key Points for Teaching

1. The goal of this lesson is to help clients use mindfulness to control their attention. It starts with the idea that pain and fear draw the mind's attention away from other things, and thus we feel more pain and fear than is effective in life. The objective is to help clients recognize when the mind is controlling their attention and mindfully choose what they will attend to and what to let go of.
2. Clients are then asked to identify "sticky" things that draw the mind's attention back away from what is effective. While it is possible that effective aspects of the situation are "sticky," this is atypical. Usually, "sticky" thoughts are ineffective and lead to rumination, obsession, judgment, or other problematic behavior. Sometimes the stickiness itself can convince the client that there is something important about the sticky thing—the way the mind comes back to it must mean it's important or worthy of attention. The goal is to help clients recognize that it is often habit or avoidance (i.e., the sticky things keep the mind from what is new or unfamiliar or fearful) that is maintaining the sticky things and it is worth repeatedly letting go of them.
3. The Opening and Refocusing the Mind handout (pp. 169–170) is all about focusing on what will be the most useful and effective aspects of a situation.
   a. Go through the in-class exercise regarding the hour before bed last night. This is a silent, guided individual exercise interspersed with discussion after the client has completed each section. Highlight that the observations the clients were most conscious of at the time (in the first step) may, in fact, have been the most effective aspects of the situation, or they may not have. The goal is deliberate and conscious observation.
   b. The refocusing of the mind step references the ideas of Thích Nhat Hanh (Hanh & Lama, 1992), which directs clients to focus on what is not wrong. Listen to the audio clip, read it out loud, or have a client do so. Ask for observations.
   c. Then return to the list of observations from the first step of the exercise and have clients consider what was happening from a Wise Mind perspective. Ask them to list what five things would have been most effective to attend to (regardless of what they actually attended to at the time).
   d. Then finally, have clients observe what the "sticky" aspects of the situation are that tend to grab and hang onto their attention, and that could trip them up when they attend to the effective aspects. Essentially, this is a troubleshooting task. Highlight how the Three Mindful Strategies taught last week can be applied to "sticky" thoughts and emotions here.
   e. If you have time, discuss clients' exercises as a group.

Presenting the Week 2 Assignment

1. Repeat the Opening and Refocusing the Mind exercise individually during a situation in which the client is having difficulty (pp. 171–172).
   a. Have the client practice considering everything happening in the present moment, and then identify what they are naturally drawn to and what, given a mindful choice, are the most effective things to think about.
   b. Then they should identify the "sticky" aspects of the situation.
   c. Ask the client to use the Three Mindful Strategies from week 1 to get unstuck and refocus on the effective things.
2. The second exercise in the Week 2 Assignment is to practice, once this week, consciously embracing what is the most important and valuable aspect of a moment they are in.
   a. They should do this for a different moment from that addressed in the previous assignment.
   b. This is less of an Observe/Describe exercise and more of a participation exercise.
   c. To this end, clients are instructed to write their observations of the experience afterward.

Reviewing the Week 2 Assignment

1. Review of these assignments can take a bit of time as it is ideal to get each client to report on each homework. If this is not possible, have different clients report on which part of the homework went particularly well or where they had questions.
2. Review daily mindfulness homework. Highlight improvements in the frequency and commitment to this compared to last week. Use commitment strategies to increase clients' commitment to practicing each day.
3. The key teaching points to highlight in the Opening and Refocusing the Mind exercise include:
   a. What differed between what the brain naturally did and what they thought would be most effective.
   b. What "sticky" thoughts interfered, and how were they able to successfully overcome the stickiness.
   c. If they weren't successful, the group can coach them on how to use the Three Mindful Strategies more effectively.
4. For the second exercise, key teaching points include:
   a. Full participation (vs. self-doubt, perfectionism, worry about the future)
   b. Accepting reality (vs. what they wish it would be) and still finding what is effective in it
   c. What was most effective might have been accompanied by positive or negative emotions (i.e., effectiveness does not always mean cheerful or pleasant)
   d. Trust in Wise Mind

Week 3: Using the Mindfulness Skills for Anxiety

Key Points for Teaching

1. The goal is twofold: Primarily, it concerns exposure to anxiety, but it is also about deepening the clients' competence with the skill of Mindfulness of Current Emotion by applying it as Mindfulness of Current Anxiety and teaching exposure.
2. Recommended reading is Chapter 14 ("Applying Mindfulness to Fear and Anxiety") from *Calming Your Anxious Mind: How Mindfulness and Compassion Can Free You from Anxiety, Fear, and Panic* by Jeffrey Brantley and Jon Kabat-Zinn (2007). This can be helpful to group leaders and clients alike if they are unfamiliar with exposure and linking mindfulness and exposure.
3. Teach the wave of emotion with SUDS rising at first (sometimes steeply) and then leveling off and gradually declining (sometimes steeply after a point). Teach how such avoidance functions to escape this process, but at the same time keeps the brain's experience of emotion as something dangerous because it is something that only increases (i.e., because the client escapes or avoids before the emotion levels off and falls).
4. Clients may experience their anxiety going off like a rocket ship that doesn't come down. This is physically impossible—the worst-case scenario of too much anxiety is failure to breathe and passing out, which stops the anxiety. The typical approach–avoidance pattern is that the person withdraws from the anxiety cue or does something else to block/reduce the anxiety. While the anxiety goes down in the short run, the brain has learned to fear the stimuli, and the anxiety will go right back up as soon as the stimuli returns again, and often more steeply.
5. Clients often feel that riding the wave is not true of them, or not true of anxiety or fear. Emphasize that the wave is a physiological reality that occurs in all humans. It may feel as if it only increases because they cut the experience off before it has its chance to peak, level, and drop off.
6. Emphasize also that a new cue will start a new wave of anxiety. If the individual brings past or future problems into the moment, they are reprompting the emotion (i.e., starting a new wave that overlaps the old). A series of overlapping waves is called a "mood" (like creating a hurricane of waves), but the original wave does not go on forever. Thus, if you can stop reprompting the event by using mindfulness of body sensations in the current moment, you can experience anxiety climbing, leveling, and falling. The goal of this week is to get the clients to experience this process by design.
7. Teach clients the concept of "corrective information." Their Emotion Mind and Wise Mind need to learn what their Reasonable Mind can see—that the situation in the current moment is not, in fact, dangerous or physically painful. The fact that a similar situation occurred in the past that was actually dangerous or physically painful does not make the current reality any more dangerous. As we know, however, Emotion Mind is not very attentive to logic, and even Wise Mind sometimes struggles. Thus, it is only the lived experience of a cue without the feared danger or pain occurring that will truly teach the correct information about what is not dangerous or physically painful.
8. We explain the difference between *in vivo* and imaginal exposure by using SDBT skills. *In*

vivo is equated to Opposite Action and imaginal exposure to Mindfulness of Current Emotion (or it can also relate to Cope Ahead). This is not an exact parallel but has been useful to our clients.

9. Highlight that exposure works best when it is "nonreinforced exposure," so the feared event does not actually occur. (Group leaders should see Foa and Rothbaum's *Treating the Trauma of Rape* [2001] for a detailed discussion of reinforced and nonreinforced exposure, if these concepts are new.) If the feared event occurs (e.g., the dog does bite you), it can make the anxiety worse, not better.
   a. In class, it helps to use examples of nonreinforced exposure like treating an elevator phobia where the elevator the person practices in falls 10 floors, or exposure for a dog phobia where the dog bites you.
   b. It may be relevant for group leaders to also consider other examples, such as flashbacks of a trauma. Often the feared event in this situation becomes so overwhelming that they reexperience the pain and horror or grow so overwhelmed that the rest of their day will be ruined or they won't sleep that night. Thus, if they practice in a situation with the trauma where they do become overwhelmed, this is nonreinforced exposure and, as happens if the dog really bites you, can make overcoming the anxiety worse. Clients should be encouraged to address this with their individual therapists if they think they might be too overwhelmed. Also, be aware the flashback example can be more subtle and some clients will get confused.
10. Highlight the other side of the dialectic that anxious people tend to believe many anxiety cues are realistic and will cause disaster. If one avoids exposing oneself to them, the anxiety will go on forever and never stop. It is important to understand enough about exposure therapy to skillfully find examples for clients to practice that are not going to be a problem without resorting to trivial anxiety cues, which won't make any real change in the client's life.
11. Clients need to be oriented that the exposure process is—more often than not—very uncomfortable. Experiencing a wave of increasing anxiety (especially when you are used to stopping it with escape or avoidance) is very stressful. It is not, however, dangerous and is probably the only path to freedom from chronic anxiety. Troubleshooting how to practice mindfulness of anxiety is not necessary in that a failure of the practice is not going to harm them. However, if troubleshooting how to practice will make it a more effective experience, more power to them.
12. It should be emphasized that having negative emotions is not a reason to avoid something. Uncomfortable things done for something you value are extremely important, and discomfort is not a reason not to do something. Sometimes it is the reason to do it. (For example, being around groups of people at softball practice week after week is very uncomfortable for socially anxious people as others often don't reach out when they are caught up in their own process or the game. One's constant presence changes the relationships all on its own, though, and people become more engaging and relationships form that wouldn't if the person didn't keep showing up.)
13. Good examples for clients to practice are events/cues that cause a midlevel SUDS peak—not so high that they lose control, but not so low as to be trivial or something they can do

now. Clients should be referred to their individual therapist for specific examples of what to practice if good examples are not quickly self-evident in group.

Presenting the Week 3 Assignment

1. Be sure to orient the group to the entire sheet for the Week 3 Assignment: Using the Mindfulness Skills for Anxiety as it takes discussion and examples to make the task clear (pp. 175–176).
2. For Daily Mindfulness, now that clients have completed different mindfulness plans in weeks 1–2, it is time for them to try staying with the same practice for the same duration, despite urges to change. This will allow them and their brains to work through any urges to avoid that naturally occur.
3. For Mindfulness of Current Anxiety, with each client, determine:
   a. How will they be mindful? What specifically will they do, when and where?
   b. How long will they practice mindfulness of their anxiety?
5. If you have doubts about their comprehension, encourage them to write notes about what is decided in group and review with their individual therapist.
6. The main part of the assignment is to set up their own Mindfulness of Current Anxiety (exposure) process, to go through the process at least once, and to write down their observations afterward.
7. This assignment is embedded with troubleshooting to maximize the likelihood of success. If you have a client expressing significant concern or distress, ask them to discuss this with their individual therapist to get individualized advice.

Reviewing the Week 3 Assignment

1. Ask for observations of practicing the same daily mindfulness practice for the same duration.
   a. If someone was unable to do so, complete a mini-chain analysis of what happened to provide guidance for next week.
   b. Reinforce willingness, participation, humor and lightness, and perseverance.
2. Ask each client to review how they approached and completed the Mindfulness of Current Anxiety (i.e., exposure) assignment.
   a. Reinforce willingness, troubleshooting, participation, bravery, and nonjudgmental observation.

Week 4: Mindfulness as a Doorway Opening to Skillful Behavior

Key Points for Teaching

1. The goal of this exercise (pp. 177–178) is to continue the application of mindfulness to more fully experience life. It builds on the themes of stopping the pattern of suppressing

emotional experience and replacing it with acceptance, interest, and learning. It is also a refinement of the Mindfulness of Current Emotion skill and general exposure principles.

2. The concepts are divided into two versions: Opening to Acceptance (practicing observing an experience then accepting it) and Opening to What Your Emotion Has to Give You (same steps adding a curious, deliberate, and kind attention to what the emotion is offering; encouraging clients to see their emotions as sources of information and strength).
3. First, highlight the importance of acceptance as the intent and outcome of this exercise. This is not about changing the moment or their experience of it; this is also not about distracting types of distress tolerance—getting through a situation by tolerating it or distracting from it—rather than mindfully participating in an experience and learning from it.
4. Start with a discussion of the goals. See if clients can generate examples of where they fight their emotions, run away from or suppress them, or get caught on the "superhighway" of their thought and rumination without getting to the heart of what is going on.
5. Then teach the Opening to Acceptance steps, which are a modification of the Mindfulness of Current Emotion skill integrated with Willingness. Practice as a group mindfulness exercise. Ask for observations and discussion.
6. Reinforce willingness, lightness, and openness.
7. Review the goals of Opening to What Your Emotion Has to Give You. Again, encourage the clients to generate examples where they hate or reject their emotions, or refuse to listen to their emotional experience.
8. Review the Opening to What Your Emotion Has to Give You steps, which start the same way as Opening to Acceptance but with two additional steps:
   a. First, clients should remind themselves that emotions are always valid (in some way). Emotions need to be accepted as present when they appear. The SDBT acceptance concept of "it is" instead of "it is OK" can be explained or reinforced.
   b. The client is then directed to "witness" their emotion—a term used specifically to imply observation, rather than participation, as well as patience and endurance. Like being with someone through a birth, a loss, an ending, or a beginning, a witness confirms what occurred; experiences it with the person; lets it happen. Like attendees at a wedding who watch the service and follow traditions of participation like the reception line—wishing the couple well but otherwise being there to observe the ritual and able to remember it with the couple afterward—even though they rarely interact directly with the couple getting married throughout the event. Thus, a witness to the emotion doesn't try to do anything with it other than offering support and being present and attentive, and remembering all of that afterward.

Presenting the Week 4 Assignment

1. The first part of the Week 4 Assignment is, again, daily mindfulness (p. 179). Note that this is the last week of daily mindfulness practice, so remind clients to stay with the practice and duration they decided on last week.
2. The other portion of the assignment is to identify situations where clients ineffectively avoid

or suppress emotions and then to practice both Opening to Acceptance and Opening to What Your Emotion Has to Give You for two such situations that arise during the week (pp. 179–181).

3. Ask for observations of hesitation or concern versus enthusiasm and willingness. Validate and highlight dialectics. Coach mindfulness tasks from weeks 1–3 as troubleshooting.

Reviewing the Week 4 Assignment

1. Ask for observations about doing 14 days of the same daily mindfulness practice and for doing a daily practice for a full month. This will be familiar to some people, but few DBT Next Steps clients have had this experience. Discuss what they learned and what, if anything, they notice at other times of the day (e.g., better sleep, easier to let things go, more relaxed).
2. Ask clients their thoughts on whether and how they might do daily mindfulness in the future. Reinforce their interest and willingness to do so.
3. Review the two Opening to Acceptance and Opening to What Your Emotion Has to Give You exercises.
4. These are the final exercises in this module, so provide specific reinforcement and feedback not only for these exercises but also for the larger concepts of living fully in the moment, mindfully experiencing pain rather than suppressing or avoiding it with rumination or distraction, and so on.

APPENDIX A

Sample Completed DBT Next Steps Skills-Training Class Notes

Date: ____________ Leaders: ______________________________

Today's topic: ______________________ Homework for next session: ____________

Client (last initial, too)	Attended? No. of misses	Homework	Any therapy-interfering behavior (BHD = no. of back homework assignments due)	Good News
Abby	On time	Done	On it. Led Check-In, upbeat and lots of GIVE skill.	
Brad	Canceled 1 miss		Emailed saying they had finals.	
Carmen	Canceled 1 miss		Emailed saying they were sick.	
Danielle	Late 10 mins	Done	Engaged.	
Eli	On time	Partial	Succeeding after DBT weeks 1 & 2.	

Check-In:

Name	Ambition	Last week's action and employment steps (note which parts are done/not done)	Action and employment steps for next week (be sure behaviorally defined)
Abby	To support myself, get out of debt and return to business I started a year ago.	Call friend who has networking group. Will call one more time if I don't hear back.	Action Step: Take my kid to the zoo. Employment Step: Attend networking group on Tuesday evening.
Brad	Complete my MSW in the next 2 years and get training in DBT afterward.		

(continued)

Sample Completed DBT Next Steps Skills-Training Class Notes *(page 2 of 2)*

Name	Ambition	Last week's action and employment steps (note which parts are done/not done)	Action and employment steps for next week (be sure behaviorally defined)
Carmen	Finish my certificate program in data management.		
Danielle	Support myself through 1 or 2 jobs, have a place, have a car, have 1–2K saved for continuing ed classes.	Try out longer work week and check in with "save my spot."	Action Step: Test drive 1 car. Employment Step: Do role-play with therapist on upcoming job interview.
Eli	Work in ideal nurse center with children, live near friends and in affordable apartment with a landlord I like.	Draft a cover letter.	Action Step: Spend 30 mins looking at housing options. Employment Step: Contact nurse colleague and ask about meeting for coffee and informational interview.
Group leader	I want to increase my organization's use of evidence-based interventions. Form CBT self-study group by end of year.	Attended Diversity, Equity, and Inclusion Committee meeting.	Employment Step: Send email to clinic about upcoming training.
Group co-leader	Defend my dissertation by the end of the year. Support a DBT training or consultation project by next year.	Scheduled meeting with advisor to discuss data analysis plan.	Employment Step: Work on dissertation for 2 hours.

APPENDIX B

Blank Template for DBT Next Steps Skills-Training Class Notes

Date: ______________ Leaders: ____

Today's topic: ____________________________ Homework for next session: ______________

Client (last initial, too)	Attended? No. of misses	Homework	Any therapy-interfering behavior (BHD = no. of back homework assignments due)	Good News

Check-In:

Name	Ambition	Last week's action and employment steps (note which parts are done/not done)	Action and employment steps for next week (be sure behaviorally defined)

(continued)

Blank Template for DBT Next Steps Skills-Training Class Notes *(page 2 of 2)*

Name	Ambition	Last week's action and employment steps (note which parts are done/not done)	Action and employment steps for next week (be sure behaviorally defined)

APPENDIX C

DBT Next Steps Pretreatment Materials

Client Application Checklist, Application Materials, and Individual and Group Therapist Performance Evaluations

DBT Next Steps Application Checklist

1. DBT Next Steps client application

☐ Review with your therapist/intake clinician to be sure you understand it.

☐ Complete on your own (often easiest to do in stages rather than all at once).

☐ Have your current therapist or the intake clinician review a draft and explain changes that are needed before you submit to team and revise accordingly.

1a. DBT Next Steps Career Plan

☐ Provide specific activities as planned throughout the DBT Next Steps year.

☐ Show how Work as Therapy and Career Development requirements will be met completely and on time.

2. DBT Individual Therapist Performance Evaluation

☐ Give Performance Evaluation form to DBT individual therapist (current or most recent) and confirm when they will complete and give to the Clinical Director.

☐ Confirm with therapist that Performance Evaluation was sent to Clinical Director.

An Individual Therapist Interim Performance Evaluation is included if you would like feedback early so you and your therapist can address any issues before the final Performance Evaluation is due (*do not turn in Interim Performance Evaluation*).

2a. DBT Skills Group Leader Performance Evaluation

☐ Give Performance Evaluation to a Skills Group leader (current or most recent) and confirm when they will complete and give to the Clinical Director.

☐ Confirm with group leader that Performance Evaluation was sent to Clinical Director.

A Group Leader Interim Performance Evaluation form is included if you would like feedback early so you and your therapist can address any issues before the final Performance Evaluation is due (*do not turn in Interim Performance Evaluation*).

3. Employment Résumé

☐ Please write (or update) a résumé that you can use for your Work as Therapy job searching that starts your first week of DBT Next Steps.

☐ Review your résumé with your therapist or intake clinician before submitting.

(continued)

DBT Next Steps Application Checklist *(page 2 of 2)*

The last two items are completed after the application and other materials are submitted to the DBT Next Steps consultation team for review.

4. DBT skills test (not included in this packet)

☐ Arrange with intake staff to take DBT skills test.

☐ Study for test.

☐ Take test (we will grade it and get you your score).

☐ If < 75% correct, develop study plan with your therapist or intake clinician.

☐ Retake exam (repeat as needed—rarely is).

5. Director/Group Leader Interview and Commitment Decision

☐ Submit application, career plan, and résumé to therapist or intake clinician.

☐ Schedule a 60-minute appointment with the Director, skills group leader, or designated clinician.

☐ Discuss interview with therapist or intake clinician to learn how to prepare.

☐ Complete interview.

☐ If steps are recommended to increase your readiness, complete them.

☐ After Director interview, review your commitment to DBT Next Steps with your current or previous therapist, or someone else whose opinion you respect, and find Wise Mind about if and when to start DBT Next Steps.

☐ Confirm with therapist or intake staff your commitment to DBT Next Steps.

When all are checked off, you are done!! Thanks for your hard work.

DBT Next Steps Client Application

Client name:	Client signature:	Date:
Therapist name:	Therapist signature:	Date:

Instructions to client: This DBT Next Steps Application Form is designed to help you focus on what you would like to achieve and what you need to do to be successful in DBT Next Steps. To start DBT Next Steps right after Standard DBT, this application must be submitted 2 months before you graduate from Standard DBT.

Section I: What Do You Want from DBT Next Steps?

1. Briefly describe your vision for a *productive working life outside mental health treatment and independent of financial support from a disability program or friends/family.* What do you aim to be doing 5 years after DBT Next Steps is over?

(continued)

2. Develop your DBT Next Steps Career Plan.

A Career Plan helps you determine your skills and interests, what career best suits your talents, and what skills and training you need for your chosen career. By developing a Career Plan, you can focus on what you want to do and how you are going to get there.

GET STARTED:

1. Decide on your career ambitions, which can help you focus more clearly on the possibilities available to you.
   a. A career ambition can be as specific as the job you want to do, such as becoming a teacher or surgeon, or can be more broad, such as being in a particular field you want to work in, for instance, education or medicine.
   b. Rather than limiting your future, a career ambition can help you discover career possibilities you wouldn't have otherwise. There are several job possibilities with any chosen career. For example, if you choose a medical career, you may want to be a pharmacy tech, scientist, nurse, or doctor.
   c. A career ambition can also guide you into doing what you want with your life—the lifestyles of scientists, nurses, and pharmacy techs are quite different (e.g., when they work, how long they work, what money they make, do they primarily lead or follow?, do they work alone or with others?, etc.).
   d. Note, write down what your Wise Mind knows now. (If you learn that you would prefer another ambition during DBT Next Steps, then it makes sense to change and you can revise your Career Plan at that time.)

2. Determine what you need to do to prepare for your chosen career. Do you need special training? If so, find out what schools offer the training you need. Also, determine what kind of experience you will need to be successful in the career. Consider an internship or volunteer work as a way to get work experience in your career field. Do you have enough emotional stamina? Do you need to save money? The answers to these questions will help you decide what your Career Activities will be.

WRITE A DETAILED PLAN in a separate document and attach the plan to this application after it is reviewed and approved by your individual therapist or the intake clinician.

Your plan should contain:
- Description of your long-term dream or ambition (e.g., 5 or 10 years from now)
- Description of the specific Career Activities you will do during the DBT Next Steps year. For each activity, specify:
  - What it is (e.g., work at *X*, class in *Y* at *Z*, etc.) Do you already have it set up? If not, include your steps to make it happen on time.
  - Time frame for it (e.g., job all year, school during fall quarter, etc.)
  - Which Recovery Goals will that activity help you achieve?

You do not have to include more than one or two activities as long as they hit the key Recovery Goals for you and make sense with your long-term ambition.

(continued)

Section II: Self-Assessment of DBT Next Steps Recovery Goals and Related Issues		
1. Please note how far you have come on each of these Recovery Goals that are the focus of DBT Next Steps. Use the following scale: 0 = Not thought about it or talked about it 1 = Thought or talked about it, no action, don't want to 2 = Thought or talked about it, no action, want to 3 = Tried to do/get it but couldn't 4 = Trying to do it, can do/have it, once or twice 5 = Trying to do it, can do/have it, not reliably 6 = Do/have this reliably, still have problems being effective 7 = Do/have this reliably, this problem is essentially solved		
Recovery Goals	**Start of DBT**	**Now**
Living Wage Employment and Off Psychiatric Disability		
Choose a Career Path to living wage employment knowing its fit with your Wise Mind values and talents, as well as the practical issues of pay, health insurance, leave and retirement benefits, hours, shift times, required training or certification, and routes to advancement.		
Demonstrate capability to financially support yourself (and your family) in your chosen career without psychiatric disability payments or partner's/family's income (if needed).		
Demonstrate capability to financially support yourself (and your family) in at least one fallback job without psychiatric disability payments or partner's/family's income (if needed).		
Have sufficient health insurance to maintain health care and medications.		
Demonstrate better than 90% follow-through at work on attendance, being on time, appropriate dress and manner, following directions, and job tasks.		
Interpersonal Proficiency		
Are interpersonally easy to work/be with—even with difficult people and during stressful times.		
Demonstrate capability to regulate emotional expression and actions, and find Wise Mind in all interpersonal situations—even with difficult people and during stressful times.		
Know your Wise Mind personal limits and act on them with yourself, employer, friends, family, colleagues, and members of your community.		
Receive praise, raises, promotions, and offers for more desirable jobs and roles within your community.		

(continued)

Recovery Goals	**Start of DBT**	**Now**
Life Outside Work *(note that these categories are expected to overlap)*		
Have at least a couple of local and/or long-distance friends whose values align with yours.		
Have at least one person or group for casual interactions (e.g., lunchroom, church, coffee, movie, book club, volunteer organization).		
Have at least one close support with whom you experience intimacy and discuss private issues (someone who is not your therapist).		
Have at least one local person or group that will notice when you are not around and would take action to find you.		
Be an active member of an organized recreational activity that is either fun or meaningful and not related to mental health (e.g., volunteer organization, church, sports teams, Spanish lessons, ballroom dancing).		
Disengage from relationships with family members that are ineffective or destructive.		
Disengage or end friendships that are ineffective or destructive.		
Choose relationships based on evidence that they are compatible with your lifestyle, needs, and values.		
Take steps to find an effective and rewarding romantic relationship (if desired).		
Emotional Proficiency		
Able to experience negative emotions building, staying, and falling mindfully—not avoiding, rushing them along, or mentally moving into a different moment.		
Able to experience positive emotions building, staying, and falling mindfully—not avoiding, rushing them along, or mentally moving into a different moment.		
Able to reduce problematic emotions effectively and fast enough to prevent them from leading to problems.		
Self-Management		
Have an effective method for managing your monthly budget and one-time expenses (e.g., new tires) so you stay within your income.		
Sufficient emergency fund savings to cover 3 months of living expenses in case you lose your job.		
Have an effective method of saving for things you would enjoy.		
Have an effective method for getting out of debt/reducing debt to a reasonable level.		
Have an effective method for managing your time that is in line with your Wise Mind values.		

(continued)

Recovery Goals	**Start of DBT**	**Now**
Have an effective method for managing your time that gets key things done on time.		
Have an effective method for managing your time that balances work, leisure, household, and downtime.		
Have an effective method of preventing illness and psychiatric symptoms from impacting your functioning.		
Develop an effective method for managing chronic illness or pain to minimize its impact on your quality of life.		

2. One of the characteristics of a life worth living outside of mental health is significant responsibilities that require time, timeliness, follow-through, patience, interest, creativity, etc. These responsibilities tend to benefit one's mental health.

	✓ if applies	
People, places, and things that I was/am responsible for/to:	**At start of DBT**	**Now**

(continued)

<table>
<tr><td colspan="5">3. What is your plan for ongoing coverage of any psychiatric medications and health issues after DBT Next Steps is completed?</td></tr>
<tr><td colspan="5">Working (or working more) may have a significant impact on your health insurance. Please become educated about your insurance before answering.</td></tr>
<tr><td colspan="5"></td></tr>
<tr><td colspan="5">What steps have you taken so far to enact this plan?</td></tr>
<tr><td colspan="5"></td></tr>
<tr><td colspan="5">Section III: Self-Assessment of DBT Next Steps Interfering Behaviors</td></tr>
<tr><td colspan="5">1. Describe the three problem behaviors that most interfere with leading a life worth living and/or reaching your vision of a productive life. Examples might include self-harm behavior/urges, substance abuse/urges, eating disorder/urges, health care overutilization, or nonadherence to medical recommendations. For each one, describe (1) the problem behavior, (2) what circumstances tend to trigger the behavior, (3) the effective strategy you are taking to increase your control over the behavior, (4) the frequency of the problem behavior at the start of DBT, and (5) the frequency of the problem behavior now.</td></tr>
<tr><td>(1) Problem behavior</td><td>(2) Circumstances that trigger</td><td>(3) Effective alternative strategy</td><td>(4) Frequency at start</td><td>(5) Frequency now</td></tr>
<tr><td></td><td></td><td></td><td></td><td></td></tr>
<tr><td></td><td></td><td></td><td></td><td></td></tr>
<tr><td></td><td></td><td></td><td></td><td></td></tr>
</table>

(continued)

2. Identify 10 judgments, assumptions, or interpretations of yourself or others that still cause you problems these days and describe the effective reframe you practice instead.	
Judgment, assumption, interpretation	**Reframe into description of situation and impact on you, self-validation**
1.	1.
2.	2.
3	3
4.	4.
5.	5.
6.	6.
7.	7.
8.	8.
9.	9.
10.	10.

3. Describe three situations or circumstances that tend to elicit willfulness that interferes with your progress toward living wage employment, social belonging, or self-management. Also describe the behavior that sometimes results from this willfulness and an effective alternative that you use. Examples include: "When I wake up feeling depressed, I sometimes get willful and think to myself 'Why bother?' and just go back to bed. Instead, I now practice the opposite action and get into the shower." "When my friend Bobby tells me I can sometimes be hard to take, I sometimes get willful and tell him off. Instead, I now practice GIVE to help Bobby feel more relaxed with me."
When . . .
. . . I sometimes . . .
. . . a more effective strategy I have been able to use instead is . . .

(continued)

When . . .
. . . I sometimes . . .
. . . a more effective strategy I have been able to use instead is . . .
When . . .
. . . I sometimes . . .
. . . a more effective strategy I have been able to use instead is . . .

4. Think about all the people in your life these days. It is likely that some of these people inadvertently reinforce your avoidance of difficult situations, avoidance that may keep you away from self-sufficiency, stuck in disability or dependence, and/or impact your ability to maintain employment or care for yourself. For example, a well-meaning friend might subtly urge you to go to the hospital instead of using skills to handle difficult feelings. A health care provider might encourage you to use more medication instead of using skills that have been effective in the past. A relative might continue paying your debt if you don't have enough money to cover it. Or a buddy might think they're helping by encouraging you to stay home from work when you are anxious, rather than finding a way to make going to work possible. These behaviors tend to be reasonable or viable only in a mental health or other dependency environment.

Describe three examples of your dependent behaviors that interfere with self-sufficiency, and how someone in your life may be inadvertently reinforcing it. Then describe what you are doing to try to reduce their problematic or ineffective influence on you.

Dependency behavior	How it's being reinforced	What I'm doing to reduce negative influence

(continued)

Dependency behavior	How it's being reinforced	What I'm doing to reduce negative influence

Section IV: Addressing Medical and Physical Limitations and Fit with DBT Next Steps
1. Describe any medical or physical difficulties or limitations you have. Include both what it is/they are as well as specific examples of how they limit your day-to-day functioning.
2. If you believe that, over the next 1–2 years, your medical or physical difficulties do or will impair your ability to work sufficiently to make a living wage so you do not need financial support from others, please describe.

(continued)

In DBT Next Steps, we have a slogan—"Contingencies create capabilities"—which is similar to the expression "Necessity is the mother of invention." This means that humans are inherently capable of more in the face of consequences. Contingencies (a.k.a. consequences) organize human behavior and focus attention toward achieving a goal. The working world makes use of this phenomenon because you get fired or lose pay if you miss work. In DBT Next Steps, we make use of the phenomenon by having requirements such as Career Activities and Work as Therapy. The consequence for not meeting a requirement is suspension from the DBT Next Steps program until that requirement is met. We are concerned that DBT Next Steps could be a poor fit for you if your medical or physical difficulties prevent you from working. Please consider and discuss with your therapist, medical provider(s), and other people you respect whether meeting DBT Next Steps contingencies is in your best interest. If this does not sound like the program for you, please work with your individual therapist to find a treatment that is a better fit or delay your application to DBT Next Steps to when your physical difficulties are resolved. If you want to pursue DBT Next Steps now and believe meeting these requirements will not negatively impact your medical or physical problems, please describe how DBT Next Steps makes sense for you.
What will you do if medical or physical difficulties arise or get worse during DBT Next Steps in order to both take care of yourself and continue in the program and meet program requirements? What strategies have worked in the past? How have you demonstrated you can and will use them?

(continued)

Section V: Addressing Treatment-Interfering Behaviors
1. Describe the steps you are taking to be more effective in health care settings. Examples might include replacing your use of emergency rooms with outpatient experts, being more direct or honest with your provider, reducing the number of health care providers you consult, or following prescribed treatments more effectively. Be as specific as possible by using frequencies (e.g., two times per month) or percentages (e.g., 15% of the time).
2. Describe three situations or circumstances that tend to elicit therapy-interfering willfulness in you. Also describe the therapy-interfering behavior that sometimes results from your willfulness and an effective alternative that you use to be more effective in therapy. Examples might include: "When my therapist asks me to assess how I came to a problem behavior, I sometimes get willful and tell her how it wasn't my fault. Now I practice radical acceptance and participation." "When my group leader asks me to get back on topic, I sometimes get willful and shut down. Now I practice GIVE; following directions with an easy manner that validates the request."
When . . .
. . . I sometimes . . .
. . . a more effective strategy I have been able to use instead is . . .
When . . .
. . . I sometimes . . .
. . . a more effective strategy I have been able to use instead is . . .

(continued)

When . . .
. . . I sometimes . . .
. . . a more effective strategy I have been able to use instead is . . .
3. Describe three additional problem behaviors that most interfere with your full participation in treatment (i.e., therapy-interfering behavior). Examples might include incomplete homework assignments, missing or late ones, being too emotionally dysregulated in session to learn effectively, or not meeting productive behavior targets. For each one, describe (1) the problem behavior, (2) what circumstances tend to trigger it, (3) the effective alternative strategy you are using instead, (4) the frequency of the problem behavior at the start of DBT, and (5) the frequency now.

(1) Problem behavior	**(2) Circumstances that trigger**	**(3) Effective alternative strategy**	**(4) Frequency at start**	**(5) Frequency now**

Thank you. You have completed the DBT Next Steps Client Application and we appreciate your thoughtfulness and willingness.

DBT Next Steps Individual Therapist Performance Evaluation

Candidate: ______________________________ Evaluation completed by: __________________

DBT start date: ___________________________ Date of this evaluation: ____________________

Purpose: The purpose of conducting this Performance Evaluation is to provide feedback to improve the quality of treatment and promote the candidate's development in preparation for DBT Next Steps as well as in social and employment settings.

Performance Rating Categories: Consider the candidate's performance in each category and designate the level that most accurately describes their performance.

- **O**—Outstanding. The candidate consistently exceeds expectations requiring little or no coaching or feedback.
- **E**—Exceeds Expectations. Results clearly exceed expectations on a regular basis. Performance is of high quality and is achieved on a consistent basis.
- **M**—Meets Expectations. Competent and dependable performance level. Meets the performance standards and objectives without constant follow-up/direction, though intermittent coaching may be needed.
- **I**—Improvement Needed/Unsatisfactory. The candidate does not meet performance expectations on a regular basis and has difficulty following through with tasks. Requires regular and consistent follow-up and/or coaching.
- **N/A**—Not applicable or too soon to rate.

General Factors

1. _____ **Quality:** The extent to which homework, Diary Cards, assignments, and work are completed thoroughly and correctly. The client is clear, prepared, and ready to participate. Challenges and pushes self in target areas. Shows a strong desire to learn and is helpful in modeling and teaching others.

   Specific Examples/Comments:

2. _____ **Independence/Reliability:** Has the ability to work independently with little or no direction, ability to complete tasks, treatment recommendations, and homework without prompting in a consistent and regular manner with consistent and regular follow-through. Minimal outside coaching is needed and able to manage difficulties between sessions on own using skills they have learned.

   Specific Examples/Comments:

(continued)

3. ______ **DBT Knowledge:** Possesses and demonstrates a thorough understanding and working knowledge of all components of DBT skills, including problem solving, reducing barriers to effective behaviors, efficient follow-through, ability to recite emotion regulation, distress tolerance, mindfulness and interpersonal effectiveness skills with minimal prompting, and shows consistent willingness and ability to generalize relevant DBT skills to necessary environments as needed in treatment, with friends and family, and across relevant social and public contexts.

   Specific Examples/Comments:

4. ______ **Interpersonal Relationships/Validation/GIVE Skills:** The extent to which the candidate is able to work and communicate well with therapists, group leaders and participants, friends, family, and others in their environment. Able to communicate effectively using active listening, validation, and compromise, while refraining from threats, judgments, and overly focusing on what they deem fair or unfair. Shows consistent ability to validate others even when they disagree and refrains from criticizing and complaining in most situations.

   Specific Examples/Comments:

5. ______ **Communication Verbal and Written:** The extent to which the candidate demonstrates clear and effective communication (includes listening, nonverbal communication, and body language) in individual and group settings across multiple contexts. Is able to make clear direct requests using DEAR MAN, describing the facts and expressing their opinions nondefensively, providing adequate reinforcement, and initiating negotiation when needed.

   Specific Examples/Comments:

6. ______ **Social Integration:** The extent to which the candidate is successfully able to adapt to and structure their environment to promote effective behavior as well as personal and social achievement. This includes adapting behavior to the social cues of those around them, ignoring others' dysfunctional behavior, and building and shaping more responsibility and/or social relationships to encourage greater success.

   Specific Examples/Comments:

(continued)

7. _____ **Leadership:** The extent to which the candidate exhibits and models effective coping, interpersonal skills, and behavior. Is able to act out of Wise Mind, being skillful, acting with integrity and confidence consistently, being interpersonally effective in clinical, education, social, and employment arenas. Is able to take initiative, frequently challenging oneself in target areas and doing more than the minimum without being prompted.

   Specific Examples/Comments:

8. _____ **Problem Identification:** The ability to troubleshoot and foresee potential barriers and problems, and develop ways to approach the situation and/or cope ahead of time with a proactive solution.

   Specific Examples/Comments:

9. _____ **Problem Solving and Decision Making:** Demonstrates ability to make sound and proper decisions by defining and identifying the problem, analyzing the causes, drawing on personal expertise and internal resources to be able to find an adequate solution. When unable to solve a problem, is able to demonstrate needed flexibility and remain on the path of effective behavior toward goals.

   Specific Examples/Comments:

10. _____ **Mental Flexibility:** The extent to which the candidate is adaptable, takes direction, goes with the flow, and can generate behavior in the service of being effective that may not be consistent with their own urges, thoughts, or emotions.

    Specific Examples/Comments:

(continued)

11. ______ **Attendance and Timeliness:** The extent to which the candidate is punctual, returns from breaks on time, and has an acceptable overall attendance record. Notifies people when running late or absent and cancels with more than 24 hours' notice, and is flexible with rescheduling. This also includes returning phone calls, emails, texts in a timely and efficient manner.

Attendance last 8 weeks: **Lateness last 8 weeks:**

Specific Examples/Comments:

Additional comments:

Areas of strength and success:

Areas in need of improvement:

DBT Next Steps Group Therapist Performance Evaluation

Candidate: ______________________________ Evaluation completed by: __________________

DBT start date: ___________________________ Date of this evaluation: ___________________

Purpose: The purpose of conducting this Performance Evaluation is to provide feedback to improve the quality of treatment and promote the candidate's development in preparation for DBT Next Steps as well as in social and employment settings.

Performance Rating Categories: Consider the candidate's performance in each category and designate the level that most accurately describes their performance.

- **O**—Outstanding. The candidate consistently exceeds expectations requiring little or no coaching or feedback.
- **E**—Exceeds Expectations. Results clearly exceed expectations on a regular basis. Performance is of high quality and is achieved on a consistent basis.
- **M**—Meets Expectations. Competent and dependable performance level. Meets the performance standards and objectives without constant follow-up/direction, though intermittent coaching may be needed.
- **I**—Improvement Needed/Unsatisfactory. The candidate does not meet performance expectations on a regular basis and has difficulty following through with tasks. Requires regular and consistent follow-up and/or coaching.
- **N/A**—Not applicable or too soon to rate.

1. ______ **Quality:** The extent to which homework, Diary Cards, assignments, and work are completed thoroughly and correctly. The client is clear, prepared, and ready to participate. Challenges and pushes self in target areas. Shows a strong desire to learn and is helpful in modeling and teaching others.

   Specific Examples/Comments:

2. ______ **Independence/Reliability:** Has the ability to work independently with little or no direction, ability to complete tasks, treatment recommendations, and homework without prompting in a consistent and regular manner with consistent and regular follow-through. Minimal outside coaching is needed and able to manage difficulties between sessions on own using skills they have learned.

   Specific Examples/Comments:

(continued)

3. _____ **DBT Knowledge:** Possesses and demonstrates a thorough understanding and working knowledge of all components of DBT skills, including problem solving, reducing barriers to effective behaviors, efficient follow-through, ability to recite emotion regulation, distress tolerance, mindfulness and interpersonal effectiveness skills with minimal prompting, and shows consistent willingness and ability to generalize relevant DBT skills to necessary environments as needed in treatment, with friends and family, and across relevant social and public contexts.

   Specific Examples/Comments:

4. _____ **Interpersonal Relationships/Validation/GIVE Skills:** The extent to which the candidate is able to work and communicate well with therapists, group leaders and participants, friends, family, and others in their environment. Able to communicate effectively using active listening, validation, and compromise, while refraining from threats, judgments, and overly focusing on what they deem fair or unfair. Shows consistent ability to validate others even when they disagree and refrains from criticizing and complaining in most situations.

   Specific Examples/Comments:

5. _____ **Communication Verbal and Written:** The extent to which the candidate demonstrates clear and effective communication (includes listening, nonverbal communication, and body language) in individual and group settings across multiple contexts. Is able to make clear direct requests using DEAR MAN, describing the facts and expressing their opinions nondefensively, providing adequate reinforcement, and initiating negotiation when needed.

   Specific Examples/Comments:

6. _____ **Social Integration:** The extent to which the candidate is successfully able to adapt to and structure their environment to promote effective behavior as well as personal and social achievement. This includes adapting behavior to the social cues of those around them, ignoring others' dysfunctional behavior, and building and shaping more responsibility and/or social relationships to encourage greater success.

   Specific Examples/Comments:

(continued)

7. _____ **Leadership:** The extent to which the candidate exhibits and models effective coping, interpersonal skills, and behavior. Is able to act out of Wise Mind, being skillful, acting with integrity and confidence consistently, being interpersonally effective in clinical, education, social, and employment arenas. Is able to take initiative, frequently challenging oneself in target areas and doing more than the minimum without being prompted.

   Specific Examples/Comments:

8. _____ **Problem Identification:** The ability to troubleshoot and foresee potential barriers and problems, and develop ways to approach the situation and/or cope ahead of time with a proactive solution.

   Specific Examples/Comments:

9. _____ **Problem Solving and Decision Making:** Demonstrates ability to make sound and proper decisions by defining and identifying the problem, analyzing the causes, and drawing on personal expertise and internal resources to be able to find an adequate solution. When unable to solve a problem, is able to demonstrate needed flexibility and remain on the path of effective behavior toward goals.

   Specific Examples/Comments:

10. _____ **Mental Flexibility:** The extent to which the candidate is adaptable, takes direction, goes with the flow, and can generate behavior in the service of being effective that may not be consistent with their own urges, thoughts, or emotions.

    Specific Examples/Comments:

(continued)

11. ______ **Attendance and Timeliness:** The extent to which the candidate is punctual, returns from breaks on time, and has an acceptable overall attendance record. Notifies people when running late or absent and cancels with more than 24 hours' notice, and is flexible with rescheduling. This also includes returning phone calls, emails, and texts in a timely and efficient manner.

Attendance last 8 weeks: **Lateness last 8 weeks:**

Specific Examples/Comments:

Additional comments:

Areas of strength and success:

Areas in need of improvement:

References

Barlow, D. H., & Craske, M. G. (2007). *Mastery of your anxiety and panic workbook* (4th ed.). Oxford University Press.

Barlow, D. H., & Craske, M. G. (2022). *Mastery of your anxiety and panic: Workbook* (5th ed.). Oxford University Press.

Blum, N., St. John, D., Pfohl, B., Stuart, S., McCormick, B., Allen, J., . . . Black, D. W. (2008). Systems Training for Emotional Predictability and Problem Solving (STEPPS) for outpatients with borderline personality disorder: A randomized controlled trial and 1-year follow-up. *American Journal of Psychiatry, 165*(4), 468–478.

Bolden, L. S., Gaona, L., McFarr, L., & Comtois, K. (2020). DBT–ACES in a multicultural community mental health setting: Implications for clinical practice. In J. Bedics (Ed.), *The handbook of Dialectical Behavior Therapy* (pp. 307–324). Academic Press.

Brantley, J., & Kabat-Zinn, J. (2007). *Calming your anxious mind: How mindfulness and compassion can free you from anxiety, fear, and panic* (2nd ed.). New Harbinger.

Carmel, A., & Comtois, K. A. (2023). Integrating dialectical behavior therapy: Accepting the challenges of employment and self-sufficiency (DBT-ACES) strategies into cognitive behavioral therapy. *Journal of Contemporary Psychotherapy: On the Cutting Edge of Modern Developments in Psychotherapy, 53*(3), 217–225.

Carmel, A., Comtois, K. A., Bolden, L. S., & McFarr, L. (2021, November 18). *A cost benefit analysis of DBT-ACES across three community mental health programs.* 26th annual ISITDBT Conference, Virtual.

Carmel, A., Comtois, K. A., Harned, M. S., Holler, R., & McFarr, L. (2016). Contingencies create capabilities: Adjunctive treatments in dialectical behavior therapy that reinforce behavior change. *Cognitive and Behavioral Practice, 23*(1), 110–120.

Chanen, A. M., Nicol, K., Betts, J. K., Bond, G. R., Mihalopoulos, C., Jackson, H. J., . . . Killackey, E. (2020). Individual Vocational and Educational Support Trial (INVEST) for young people with borderline personality disorder: Study protocol for a randomised controlled trial. *Trials, 21*(583).

Comtois, K. A., Carmel, A., McFarr, L. M., Höeschel, K., Huh, D., Murphy, S., . . . Höeschel, S. (2020).

DBT—Accepting the Challenges of Employment and Self-Sufficiency (DBT-ACES) effectiveness: A re-evaluation in three settings. *DBT Bulletin, 1*(3), 14–23. https://cbtcalifornia.com/wp-content/uploads/2020/06/DBT-Bulletin_Vol3Iss1_June-2020.pdf

Comtois, K. A., Elwood, L., Holdcraft, L. C., Smith, W. R., & Simpson, T. L. (2007). Effectiveness of dialectical behavior therapy in a community mental health center. *Cognitive and Behavioral Practice, 14*(4), 406–414.

Comtois, K. A., Kerbrat, A. H., Atkins, D., Harned, M., & Elwood, L. (2010). Recovery from disability for individuals with borderline personality disorder: A feasibility trial of DBT-ACES. *Psychiatric Services, 61*(11), 1106–1111.

Comtois, K. A., Koons, C. R., Kim, S. A., Manning, S. Y., Bellows, E., & Dimeff, L. A. (2007). Implementing standard dialectical behavior therapy in an outpatient setting. In L. A. Dimeff & K. Koerner (Eds.), *Dialectical behavior therapy in clinical practice: Applications across disorders and settings* (pp. 37–68). Guilford Press.

Cook, J. A., Lehman, A. F., Drake, R., McFarlane, W. R., Gold, P. B., Leff, H. S., . . . Grey, D. D. (2005). Integration of psychiatric and vocational services: A multisite randomized, controlled trial of supported employment. *American Journal of Psychiatry, 162*(10), 1948–1956.

Cunningham, K., Wolbert, R., & Lillie, B. (2004). It's about me solving my problems: Clients' assessments of dialectical behavior therapy. *Cognitive and Behavioral Practice, 11*(2), 248–256.

Department of Social Services, Australian Government. (n.d.). *Disability Support Pension (DSP) eligibility and evidentiary.* www.dss.gov.au/disability-and-carers-benefits-payments/disability-support-pension-dsp-eligibility-and-evidentiary

Dimeff, L. (2014) Questions to ask when picking a DBT program. Portland DBT Institute. http://pdbti.org/wp-content/uploads/2014/10/Questions-to-ask-when-picking-a-DBT-program.pdf

Drake, R. E., & Deegan, P. E. (2008). Are assertive community treatment and recovery compatible? Commentary on "ACT and recovery: Integrating evidence-based practice and recovery orientation on assertive community treatment teams." *Community Mental Health Journal, 44*(1), 75–77.

Drake, R. E., McHugo, G. J., Bebout, R. R., Becker, D. R., Harris, M., Bond, G. R., & Quimby, E. (1999). A randomized clinical trial of supported employment for inner-city patients with severe mental disorders. *Archives of General Psychiatry, 56*(7), 627–633.

Foa, E. B., Hembree, E., & Rothbaum, B. (2007). *Prolonged Exposure Therapy for PTSD: Emotional processing of traumatic experiences, therapist guide.* Oxford University Press.

Foa, E. B., & Rothbaum, B. C. (2001). *Treating the trauma of rape: Cognitive-behavioral therapy for PTSD.* Guilford Press.

Gold, P. B., Meisler, N., DuRoss, D., & Bailey, L. (2004). Employment outcomes for hard-to-reach persons with chronic and severe substance use disorders receiving Assertive Community Treatment. *Substance Use and Misuse, 39*(13–14), 2425–2489.

Gold, P. B., Meisler, N., Santos, A. B., Carnemolla, M. A., Williams, O. H., & Keleher, J. (2006). Randomized trial of supported employment integrated with Assertive Community Treatment for rural adults with severe mental illness. *Schizophrenia Bulletin, 32*(2), 378–395.

Government of Canada. (2015, October 14). *Canada Pension Plan disability benefits: Do you qualify* [Service initiation]. www.canada.ca/en/services/benefits/publicpensions/cpp/cpp-disability-benefit/eligibility.html

Hanh, T. N., & Dalai Lama, H. H. (1992). *Peace is every step: The path of mindfulness in everyday life* (A. Kotler, Ed.). Random House.

Horvitz-Lennon, M., Reynolds, S., Wolbert, R., & Witheridge, T. F. (2009). The role of Assertive Community Treatment in the treatment of people with borderline personality disorder. *American Journal of Psychiatric Rehabilitation, 12*(3), 261–277.

Katsakou, C., Marougka, S., Barnicot, K., Savill, M., White, H., Lockwood, K., & Priebe, S. (2012).

Recovery in borderline personality disorder (BPD): A qualitative study of service users' perspectives. *PLoS ONE, 7*(5), e36517.

Linehan, M. (1993). *Cognitive-behavioral treatment of borderline personality disorder.* Guilford Press.

Linehan, M. (2025a). *DBT skills training handouts and worksheets* (rev. ed.). Guilford Press.

Linehan, M. (2025b). *DBT skills training manual* (rev. ed.). Guilford Press.

Markowitz, J. C., Bleiberg, K., Pessin, H., & Skodol, A. E. (2007). Adapting interpersonal psychotherapy for borderline personality disorder. *Journal of Mental Health, 16*(1), 103–116.

McCann, R. (n.d.). *Mindfulness practices—Shoe mindfulness.* Treatment Implementation Collaborative. www.ticllc.org/mindfulness-practices

Morgenstern, J. (n.d.). *WorkSMART solutions: Create a culture of productivity and wellbeing.* www.juliemorgenstern.com

Morgenstern, J. (2004). *Time management from the inside out: The foolproof system for taking control of your schedule—and your life* (2nd ed.). Henry Holt/Owl Books.

Pryor, K. (2018). *Don't shoot the dog: The new art of teaching and training.* Ringpress.

Sarafino, E. P. (2011). *Self-management: Using behavioral and cognitive principles to manage your life.* Wiley.

Schmidt, J., Lu, T., Boyle, T., & Vedantam, S. (2018). *When everything clicks: The power of judgment-free learning* [Podcast]. www.npr.org/2018/06/04/616127481/when-everything-clicks-the-power-of-judgment-free-learning

Social Security Administration. (n.d.). How do we define disability? In *The Red Book* (SSA Publication No. 64-030). www.ssa.gov/redbook/eng/definedisability.htm?tl=0

Swenson, C. R., Torrey, W. C., & Koerner, K. (2002). Implementing dialectical behavior therapy. *Psychiatric Services, 53*(2), 171–178.

Tsai, M., Kohlenberg, R. J., Kanter, J. W., Holman, G., & London, M. P. (2012). *Functional analytic psychotherapy.* Routledge.

Weisbrod, B. A. (1983). A guide to benefit-cost analysis, as seen through a controlled experiment in treating the mentally ill. *Journal of Health Politics, Policy and Law, 7*(4), 808–845.

Wolpe, J. (1969). *Subjective Units of Distress Scale* [Dataset].

Wolpe, J. (1990). *The practice of behavior therapy* (4th ed.). Pergamon Press.

Index

Note. *f* or *t* following a page number indicates a figure or a table.

D

E

T

U

V

W